THE BRAIN

AND CENTRAL NERVOUS SYSTEM

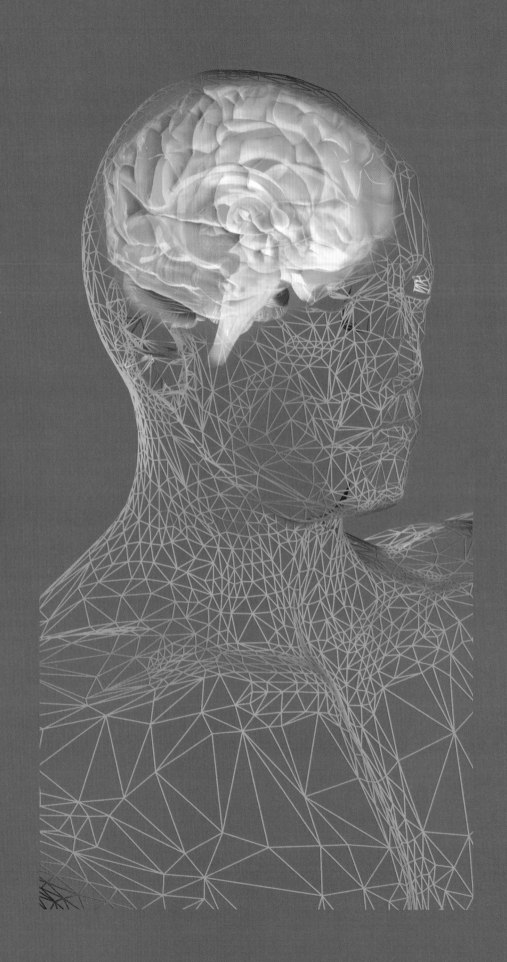

B R THE A I N

AND CENTRAL NERVOUS SYSTEM

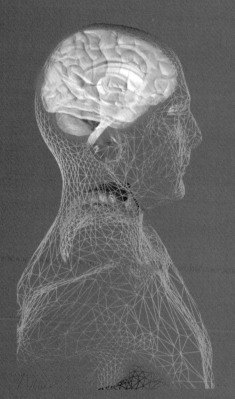
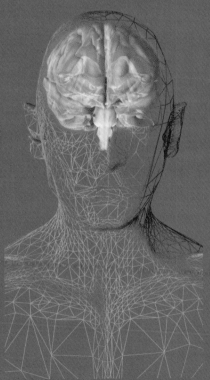
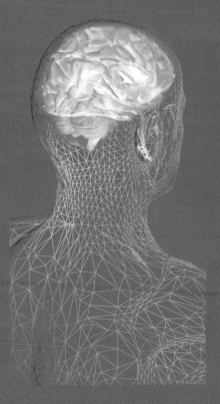

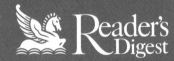
Reader's Digest

The Reader's Digest Association, Inc.

Pleasantville, New York

London Sydney Montreal

The Brain and Central Nervous System

was created and produced by
Carroll & Brown Limited
20 Lonsdale Road
London NW6 6RD

Library of Congress Cataloging-in-Publication
Data has been applied for.

ISBN 0-7621-0436-8

Printed in the United States of America
1 3 5 7 9 8 6 4 2

The information in this book is for
reference only; it is not intended as a
substitute for a doctor's diagnosis and
care. The editors urge anyone with
continuing medical problems or
symptoms to consult a doctor.

American Edition Produced by

NOVA Graphic Services, Inc.
501 Office Center Drive, Suite 190
Ft. Washington, PA 19034 USA
(215)542-3900

President
David Davenport

Editorial Director
Robin C. Bonner

Composition Manager
Steve Magnin

Art Director
Karen Kappe

Neurology Specialist Consultant
Dr. Lesley Fellows, MDCM, DPhil, Center for Cognitive Neuroscience,
University of Pennsylvania

CONTRIBUTORS

Dr Catrin Blank, BSc, MBBS, MRCP, Imperial College London

Dr Francesca Crawley, BA, MB ChB, MRCP, MD, Department of Neurology,
Charing Cross Hospital, London

Dr Adrienne Key, MB ChB, MRCPsych Department of Psychiatry,
St George's Hospital Medical School, London

Joel Levy, BSc, MA, Freelance medical writer

Sheila Merriman, SRD, FRSH, DipAPD, RNutr, Head of Nutrition and Dietitic Service,
St Andrew's Hospital, Northampton

Dr Ivan Moseley, MD, PhD, FRCP, Department of Neuroradiology,
National Hospital for Neurology and Neurosurgery, London

Mr Kevin O'Neill, BSc, MBBS, FRCS (SN), Department of Neurosurgery,
Charing Cross Hospital, London

Nageena Rahman, BPharm, MRPharmS, Drug Information Pharmacy Department,
Charing Cross Hospital, London

Dr Andrew Scholey, BSc, PhD, CPsychol, AFBTFS, Human Cognitive Neuroscience Unit,
Division of Psychology, University of Northumbria

Dr Jeremy Stern, BMA, MB BChir, MRCP, DHMSA, Medical Research Council, London

Mr Christian Ulbricht, BSc, MBBS, FRCS, Department of Neurosurgery,
Charing Cross Hospital, London

Dr Richard P White

Amanda Wright, MCSP MSc, Physiotherapy Department, King's College London

For the Reader's Digest
Editor in Chief Neil E. Wertheimer
Editorial Director Christopher Cavanaugh
Senior Designer Judith Carmel
Production Technology Manager Douglas A. Croll
Manufacturing Manager John L. Cassidy

The Brain and Central Nervous System

Awareness of health issues and expectations of medicine are greater today than ever before. A long and healthy life has come to be looked on as not so much a matter of luck but as almost a right. However, as our knowledge of health and the causes of disease has grown, it has become increasingly clear that health is something that we can all influence, for better or worse, through choices we make in our lives. *Your Body Your Health* is designed to help you make the right choices to make the most of your health potential. Each volume in the series focuses on a different physiological system of the body, explaining what it does and how it works. There is a wealth of advice and health tips on diet, exercise and lifestyle factors, as well as the health checks you can expect throughout life. You will find out what can go wrong and what can be done about it, and learn from people's real-life experiences of diagnosis and treatment. Finally, there is a detailed A to Z index of the major conditions that can affect the system. The series builds into a complete user's manual for the care and maintenance of the entire body.

This volume looks at the body's control center—the brain and central nervous system. If your brain controls your body, then what controls your brain? This is just one of the many questions answered in this fascinating account of the anatomy and health of the brain, which takes you from the microscopic details of nerve cells to the physical, emotional, and intellectual functions controlled by different parts of the brain. Find out why memory and other functions respond so characteristically to an alcoholic beverage or two. Discover which foods can combat stress and how to eat to beat depression. We're all losing brain cells at an astonishing rate, but a regular brain workout can help you live better longer. Meet the brain doctors and find out how they work out what's wrong—from simply watching how a person walks to advanced technologies that let them see what's inside our heads. And read about the range of available treatments, from drug therapy to life-saving brain surgery.

Contents

1

How your brain works

2

Brain-healthy living

TAKE CHARGE OF YOUR BRAIN HEALTH

LIVE A BRAIN-HEALTHY LIFESTYLE

EAT A BRAIN-HEALTHY DIET

STIMULATE YOUR BRAIN

3

What happens when things go wrong

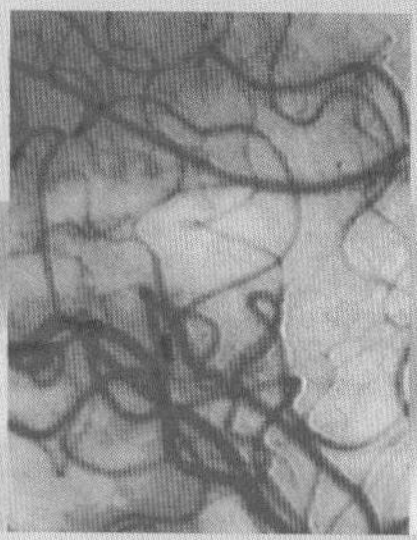

The life story of the brain

Do you know what is going on inside your head? If you answered yes, think again—even the world's foremost brain scientists would find it hard to make this claim. After more than a century of study, many aspects of the brain's functions are still mysterious. Every answer that scientists find raises new questions, while the central riddles of the brain—about consciousness and the mind—remain unsolved.

Every second of every day, a constant blizzard of mental activity rages through your brain. You are only aware of the uppermost levels of this storm—the thoughts, ideas and perceptions that make up your consciousness. Below these, lies an invisible whirl of activity—the enigmatic world of the unconscious.

As you read these lines, a host of mental processes is going on simultaneously in your head. A fraction of an inch in from the base of your skull, a tiny patch of brain tissue is telling your heart how fast to beat. As your eye tracks along the line, a whole chain of brain cells fires in concert to control and coordinate your eye muscles. You decide to turn the page—within a fraction of a second, your brain sends precise instructions to the muscles of your fingers, hand, arm, and shoulder. These are remarkable abilities, but your brain is capable of so much more. For instance, as you read this text, signals race across the surface of your brain, interpreting the marks on the page as words, giving each of them meaning and putting them together to make sentences. You glance at the picture below, and it reminds you of something—images and sounds received long ago are retrieved from storage and come to life in your imagination. Perhaps most mysterious of all, your brain lets you think about what it is doing as it's doing it: You are capable of self-reflection, of thinking about thinking.

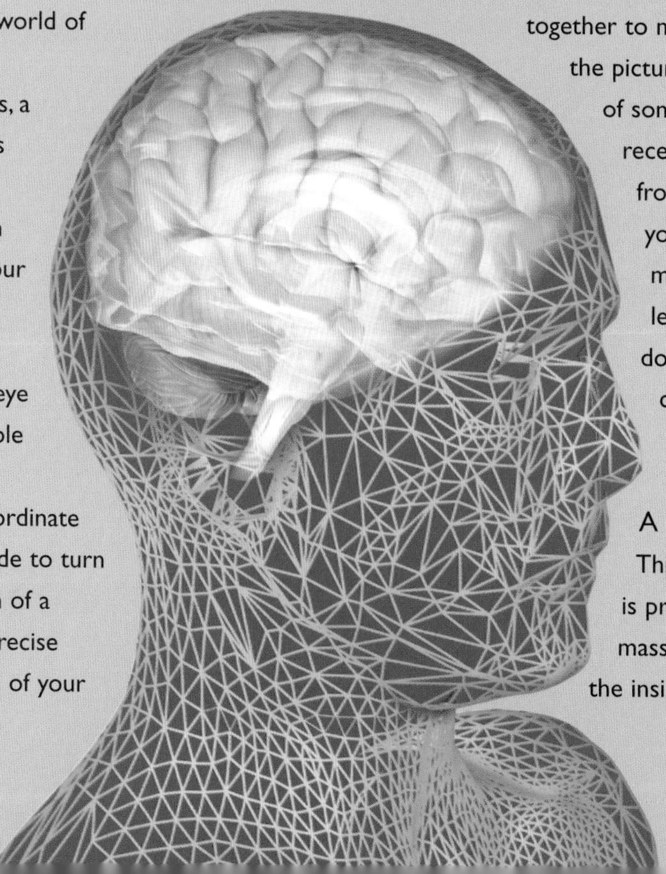

A BRAIN OF SUBSTANCE

This astonishing range of activity is produced by an unprepossessing mass of pinkish-gray tissue that fills the inside of your skull (the brain) and extends down your back to just below your waist in the spinal cord. Together, brain and spinal cord are known as the central nervous system and are responsible for collecting, processing, and responding to information from nerves all over the body and, via the senses, from the world outside. The brain is the larger part of the system. On average it weighs about 3 pounds, which may not sound like much, yet the brain is the central feature of human evolution and the key to our success as a species.

What makes the human brain such a remarkable piece of mental equipment, and how did we get it? The fossil record of human evolution is sketchy, but researchers have found that the most profound change has been in the size of the brain. Brain capacity went from about 22 ounces in the 1.9-million-year-old hominid *Homo habilis*, to about 32 ounces in *Homo erectus* (1.5 million years ago), to a whopping 47 ounces in *Homo sapiens* today. One particular part of the brain grew bigger than in any other animal—the outer layer, known as the cerebrum, which is the most obvious and striking feature of the human brain. The cerebrum is convoluted and folded to fit as much of it as possible into the skull, and it is the development of this large cerebrum that provided the crucial boost to human intelligence.

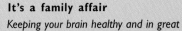

It's a family affair
Keeping your brain healthy and in great mental shape has a lot to do with your family medical history: whether or not a particular condition runs in your family.

The human brain is packed with more than 100 billion nerve cells, roughly the same as the number of trees in the Amazon rain forest. Brain activity involves nerve cells talking to one another via connections called synapses. The more synapses there are, the more communication there is and the more powerful your brain becomes. What makes the human brain so utterly remarkable is the number of connections it contains—around 100 trillion. Even more incredible, this represents just the tip of an enormous iceberg; as you learn and develop, you make new connections, so that every new experience subtly alters the arrangement of synapses in your brain.

A BRAIN AS INDIVIDUAL AS YOU ARE

This amazing complexity is arranged into a pattern unique to your individual consciousness—the pattern that makes up your personality, intelligence, memories, and thoughts. What determines this pattern? What decides whether your particular 100 billion nerve cells combine to make you a happy person or a sad one, an aggressive or gentle one, or

You have at least 100 trillion connections (synapses) in your brain— that's 100,000,000,000,000! This is greater than the estimated number of leaves on the trees in the Amazon rain forest.

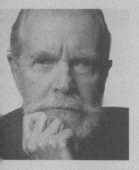

an intelligent or slow one? The search for an answer to this question has sparked a fierce debate that has raged since brain research was in its infancy—the nature–nurture debate.

On the nurture side of this fundamental divide are those who argue that upbringing is everything, and that your environment is what shapes your brain and therefore your personality. On the other side are those who contend that you would have turned out much the same whether you had been raised in a cabin in Alaska or a towerblock in Hanoi. They would argue that your personality is determined mainly by the genes you inherit from your parents. It is this latter group who are gaining ground in the field of brain research today, as new techniques allow them to probe the secrets of the human genetic code and attempt to match genes with personality characteristics such as alcoholism or depressive tendencies. More and more discoveries of this kind are being made, although the picture is usually far more complicated than the media would have you believe. Discovering a gene "for" a particular trait usually means that researchers have found only one of many possible genes that may be involved, and that the gene merely gives rise to a predisposition to the trait.

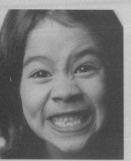

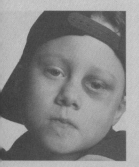

Nonetheless, this research offers both exciting and disturbing possibilities for the future. For instance, it may soon be possible to screen patients with depression

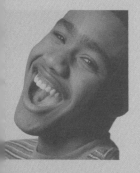

There's no one quite like you
Even though every brain is made from the same component parts, everyone is different.

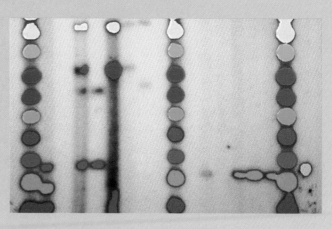

DNA sequencing
Sophisticated techniques, such as genetic fingerprinting, can identify whether a person carries the genes that may put them at risk for a neurological condition, for example Tay–Sachs disease.

to see if they are at particularly high risk of suicide. If so, they could be targeted for intensive life-saving treatment. On the otherhand, people who tested positive, say, for a gene that predisposes them for alcoholism, may never touch a drop in their lives, but could be denied various types of employment on the basis of a genetic accident.

STARTING OUT

The unique pattern of your brain is determined by the interaction of genes and experience. Even as a baby's brain forms in the womb, this interaction is shaping and molding the growing mass of cells. The fact that human brains are created by a combination of processes is another massive evolutionary advance, as important as the overall increase in brain size. To understand what this means, imagine the human brain during fetal and childhood development as a canvas, with a unique shape created by genetic inheritance, ready for experience and learning to paint it. By comparison, the brains of other animals are much smaller canvases, almost fully formed at birth, on which only the roughest sketches can be drawn by experience. Whereas animals are restricted by instinct and capable of only limited learning, humans can develop language, reasoning, social skills, and imagination.

The story of how this "canvas" is formed is one of the most incredible episodes in the human life cycle. It begins

At the peak of fetal brain growth, 250,000 new nerve cells are being produced every minute (15 million an hour).

with a few cells at one end of a tiny embryo and builds into the collection of billions of nerve cells that make up the adult brain and spinal cord. At the beginning, of course, is the fertilized egg. Within a week, rapid division has transformed this single cell into a ball of hundreds of cells, which quickly organizes itself into a head and a "tail" end, and a front and back. By week 3, there is a groove along the back of the tiny embryo; the lips of this groove meet and fuse to form a 1⁄17-inch-long neural tube. From this tube the spinal cord, nerves, and brain will develop.

By week 4, the head end of the neural tube is starting to swell, and has already split into different regions. The very top, where the cerebrum will develop, grows fastest. At week 5 it is noticeably swollen, and lower portions of the neural tube have become the spinal cord and are

sprouting nerves. By week 8, the cerebrum is the dominant feature of the embryonic brain. Below it, the lower portions of the brain begin to bend and flex, swelling and enveloping one another, becoming the structures called the brainstem and cerebellum.

Inside these regions, cells are dividing at a frantic rate. These cells move around, migrating to different parts of the brain and spinal cord, sending out feelers and tentacles to make contact with one another. They organize themselves into the patterns that turn their random electrical activity into perceptions and thoughts. After week 9, the developing baby is called a fetus. Between weeks 9 and 12 the brain and nerves start to function, and by week 20, when the fetus is about 7½ inches long, it can react to sounds from the outside world.

AN INCREDIBLE JOURNEY

Your central nervous system is one of the first systems of the body to develop. By week 3, the cells that form the basis of the brain and spinal cord—the neural tube—are already visible.

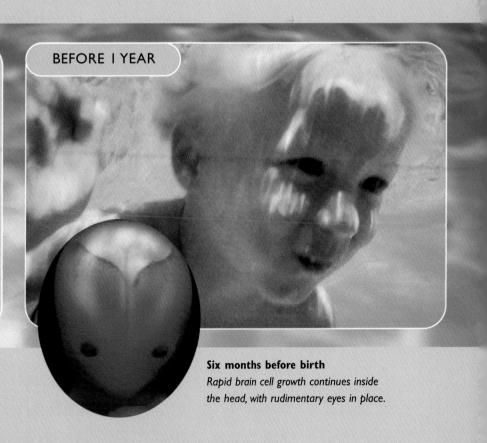

BEFORE I YEAR

Six months before birth
Rapid brain cell growth continues inside the head, with rudimentary eyes in place.

SHAPING THE BRAIN FOR LIFE

A baby is born with as many nerve cells as he or she will ever have. In the following years, individual cells will enlarge, and the masses of support cells that keep your brain running smoothly will grow, but the number of nerve cells will inexorably decline. Most of this decline happens right away. Within the first year, half of the nerve cells are pruned away, as the brain is literally sculpted into shape. At the same time, billions of connections are forged, broken, and reforged between the nerve cells. Children's brains are rewired on a massive scale as they soak up information from the environment, learning complex skills such as language at a speed beyond the capabilities of any adult.

Around the age of seven, brain cells undergo a process called myelination, which acts to fix nerve pathways in place but in doing so restricts their capacity to change and adapt. Myelination provides a sort of physiological rationale for the famous Jesuit maxim "Give me a child until the age of seven, and I will give you the man."

Recent research has found what most parents already know—that teenagers' brains are different from everyone else's. Neuroscientists in the United States and Canada have found evidence that suggests an anatomical explanation for the behavior that exasperates parents. It seems that vital sections of the cerebrum expand at the beginning of puberty and then shrink as the brain reaches adulthood. The frontal and parietal lobes, which are responsible for activities such as planning and self-control, go through a growth spurt around the age of 12. Then, in a process similar to that of the massive nerve cell decline of

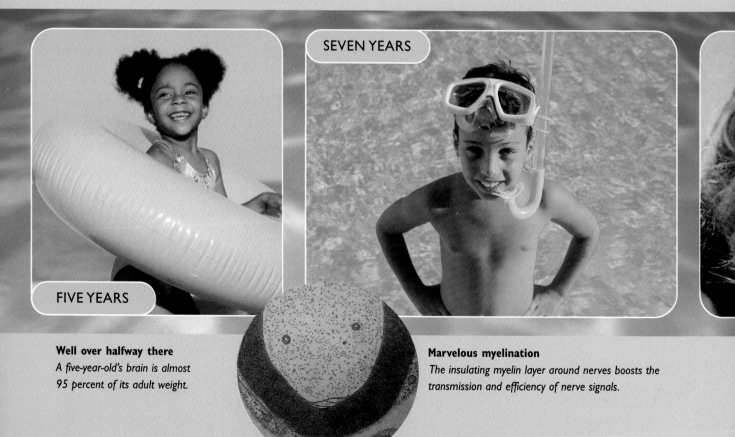

SEVEN YEARS

FIVE YEARS

Well over halfway there
A five-year-old's brain is almost 95 percent of its adult weight.

Marvelous myelination
The insulating myelin layer around nerves boosts the transmission and efficiency of nerve signals.

early childhood, the cells in these areas are pruned into a pattern that fits the adolescent brain for the complexities of life as an independent adult.

Teenage brainstorms notwithstanding, your brain has looked much the same since you were a child. The adolescent developments just described involve very small changes in the thickness of the cerebrum. Maturation in the brain generally involves modifications in the number and pattern of synapses, changes that are barely visible even on a microscopic scale. By late adulthood, you are shedding over 100,000 brain cells a day, simply as a result of normal wear and tear. You lose about 7 percent of your brain cells over the course of your adult life. By the time you reach extreme

old age, a few changes will have taken place. The outer layer of the cerebrum, called the cortex, thins out slightly, and fluid-filled spaces in your brain called ventricles (which help to nourish and support the brain tissue) enlarge.

Neither of these developments has much impact on brain power. Much more serious is the deterioration in the blood supply to your brain. Nerve cells are energy hungry, and the brain is equipped with a rich blood supply. As you age, blood vessels all over your body become less elastic, and deposits (of plaque) build up inside them, restricting blood flow and making them ever more vulnerable to blockage by blood clots or debris.

Reduced blood supply means reduced brain power, and blockage of even a tiny blood vessel in the brain can cause a significant area of tissue to die. This is

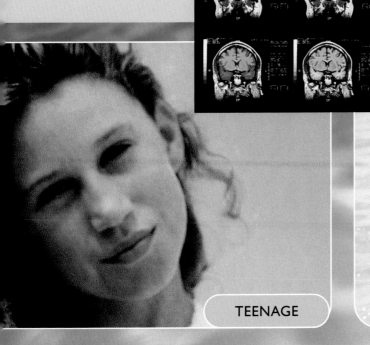

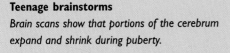

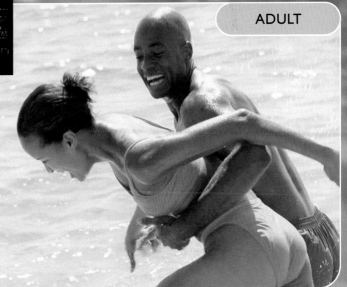

ADULT

Teenage brainstorms
Brain scans show that portions of the cerebrum expand and shrink during puberty.

Grown-up stability
Barring disease or damage, your brain will look much the same throughout adult life, despite the fact that cells are continually lost.

called a stroke. Large strokes have catastrophic consequences and are one of the leading causes of death in Western society. More common are tiny strokes, not even noticed at the time, that cause progressive build-up of damage and decline in brain function.

SAFEGUARD YOUR BRAIN HEALTH

In the developed world an increasing proportion of the population is living longer, so age-related issues are becoming more important. Skyrocketing rates of Alzheimer's disease (an estimated 14 million Americans may be afflicted by 2050) have sparked anxieties about "gray plagues." Meanwhile, economists issue warnings about the proportion of GDP that will be expended on medicare and nursing home expenses.

OLDER PEOPLE

Protecting against age-related risks
As you age, it is vital to look after your heart to reduce the risk of stroke from a clot blocking a vital blood vessel in the brain.

Being aware of both the importance and the vulnerability of your brain is essential. Taking charge of the health of your central nervous system and adopting a "brain-friendly" lifestyle can pay enormous dividends in terms of quality of life: a longer and healthier old age, greater mental energy and vitality, a better memory, and a more active and fulfilling role in the community. Achieving these benefits depends on a few key elements, such as adopting a simple program of health checks, eating a balanced diet, getting regular exercise, not smoking, learning how to deal with stress, and keeping mentally active.

When things do go wrong, medical science is increasingly equipped to help out. The last decades have seen radical advances in the diagnosis and understanding of nervous system–related health issues. New imaging techniques, such as MRI and CT scanning, have enabled doctors and scientists to view the living brain and to pinpoint problems with great accuracy. Drug therapies and surgical treatment options now exist for a wide range of physical and mental problems, and the future promises some amazing possibilities.

THE FUTURE LOOKS BRIGHT

Biotechnology is often in the headlines, especially with such feats of modern science as cloning and genetic engineering. The application of these technologies to the development of new therapies will happen in the near future. Scientists will be able to produce new nerve cells from patients' own tissues and use them to repair brain damage and diseases such as Parkinson's. Brain grafts may even be able to help treat Alzheimer's or to repair the normal wear and tear of aging, turning back the clock and rejuvenating old brains.

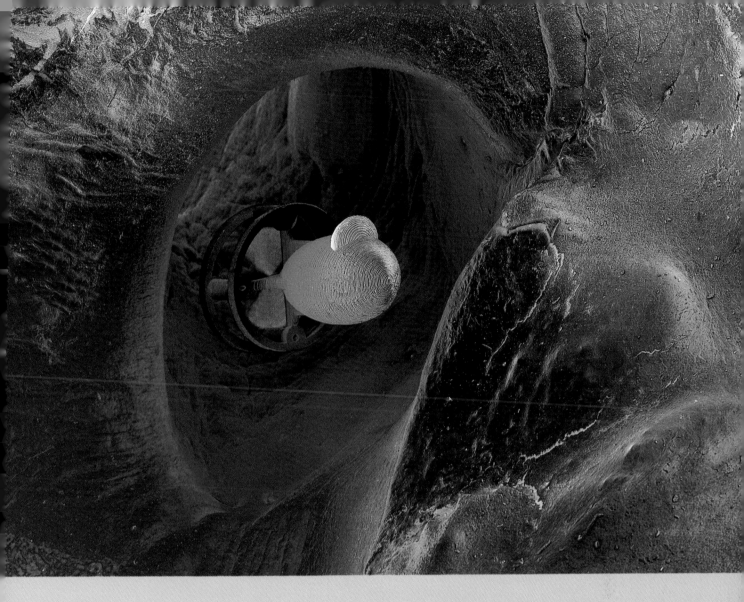

Gene therapy involves changing the genetic code of a living person. Its most obvious application, which is already being tested around the world, is in the treatment of disorders caused by straightforward genetic errors, such as Huntington's chorea, but more complex treatments are also being tested—the year 2001 saw gene therapy trials for Alzheimer's. In the future, gene therapy may be used to treat cancer, cardiovascular problems that cause strokes, or mental illness such as schizophrenia.

Looking further ahead, predictions enter the realm of science fiction, but inventors and engineers are already actively working toward fundamental changes in the way we think about ourselves. In 1999, the first cybernetic eye was wired into the brain of a man who has been blind from birth. Photosensors in a special pair of glasses pick up light and feed it into a computer that is connected directly to his brain, giving him the ability to "see" rough

Nanosubmarines may keep us alive
Sometime in the near future, micromolecular machines—nanorobots or nanosubmarines (shown above, as one would look in a blood vessel)—will blast plaques or clots within blood vessels to reduce the risk of a stroke and the consequent brain damage.

shapes and shades. Relatively soon there could be more complete integration of information technology and the brain. Humans could well have microchips wired into their nervous systems, augmenting their natural abilities and giving direct mental access to the computer world. Such developments could radically redefine what it means to be human. But how can something as fundamental as our humanity be altered? The answer lies in that remarkable tangle of cells that sits inside your head, governing your every movement, from the beating of your heart to the twiddling of your thumbs—it is your amazing brain.

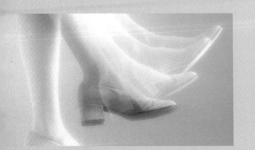 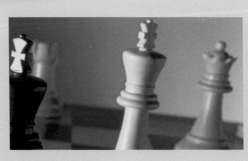 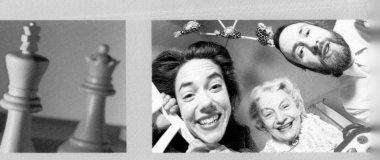

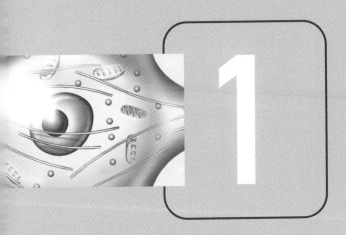

1

How your brain works

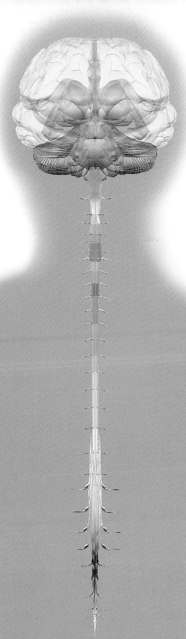

Your amazing central nervous system

As the master controller of your body, your central nervous system—your brain and spinal cord—oversees and coordinates your inner world, while enabling you to make sense of the world outside.

EXPLORING THE CENTRAL NERVOUS SYSTEM

Your brain and spinal cord form your central nervous system, the most amazing, complex and exciting set of tissues in your body. In the following pages, we will look at how these delicate and vital structures are protected; then we get down to the basics of explaining neurons—the nerve cells that form the building blocks not just of the brain, but of the entire nervous system. From all around your body, nerve cells build into nerve bundles, which join together to relay information and carry instructions. They gather at your spine, where they connect with a column—the spinal cord—that ascends to your brain.

Where the cord meets the brain, a series of bulges marks the first primitive parts of the brain—the brainstem and cerebellum. Further on, this stem abruptly swells into a large mass with a surface resembling a walnut, marked by deep grooves and ridges—this is the cerebrum, a complex part of the brain with many diverse functions. We finish our journey through the brain with a look at the unconscious mechanisms that control your brain over the course of a typical day as you cope with the challenges of everyday life.

One neuron may be linked to as many as 50,000 others; the brain is estimated to contain over 100 trillion connections. The total number of possible connections is higher than the number of atoms in the universe.

What happens where?
Certain functions, such as speech, have been traced to particular areas of the brain. Discover which part of your brain controls which part of your body on pages 34 to 41.

The cerebellum *is pivotal in the coordination of your body's movements. It forms one of the basic divisions of the brain; see pages 28 to 29.*

The cerebrum *controls all our conscious thoughts and actions—the abilities (such as language; see page 40) and qualities that make us human and give us our identities.*

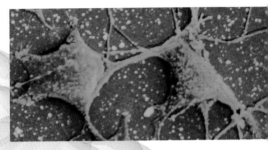

From neuron to nerve bundle
There are 100 billion nerve cells—neurons— in your brain. Everything you see, feel, think and do depends on their ability to communicate with each other. Find out how they do this and how they join together to form nerves on pages 22 to 25.

Ventricles *are fluid-filled spaces within your brain with an essential protective function; see pages 20 to 21.*

The brainstem *controls the most basic unconscious processes of your body, such as your blood pressure, and breathing and heart rates; see pages 28 to 29.*

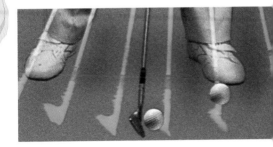

Anyone for a game of golf?
To make the movements of a simple golf swing, your brain not only has to do complex mathematics to judge distance and force but also has to work to keep you balanced and upright. Find out how it does this on pages 36 to 37.

The limbic system *is a primitive brain structure that governs hunger, sex drive, and your emotions. Find out more on pages 30 to 31.*

Protection and support

For protection from physical injury and the "invisible" world of infection, as well as for weightless support, the brain and spinal cord employ a three-line defense of bone, specialized membranes, and a unique fluid.

CRASH HELMET AND SHOCK ABSORBER

The brain and spinal cord are encased in bony structures, which provide external protection. But the delicate tissue inside must also be protected from contact or impact with the bone itself, and it is the job of three membranes known as the meninges to take on this shock-absorbing role. They work together with a unique liquid, the cerebrospinal fluid (CSF), to protect and support the brain cells and nerves of the spinal cord.

Floating in fluid

Spaces within the brain called ventricles secrete CSF at a rate of about 1 tbsp (15 ml) per hour. This clear, colorless liquid fills the ventricles and flows around the outside of the brain and down the spinal cord, bathing the entire central nervous system in a protective and nourishing fluid coating. Together with the meninges, CSF cushions your brain's movement inside the skull, whether you suffer a serious accident or simply bump into a lamppost.

Holes in the head

Enlarged ventricles are a tell-tale sign of degenerative diseases such as Alzheimer's or of damage caused by alcoholism. As brain tissue shrinks, the fluid-filled ventricles expand to take up the empty space, so that they appear abnormally large as shown here in yellow on this brain scan of a person with Alzheimer's disease; the normal size is drawn in pink. Ventricles also dramatically increase in size in a rare condition called hydrocephalus. In this disorder, the ventricles over-secrete CSF and expand to accommodate the extra fluid. Neurosurgeons insert a long, thin tube from the ventricles into the abdominal cavity, where the excess CSF is reabsorbed by the body.

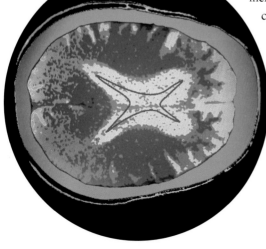

The skull is the hard, bony "crash helmet" that provides protection on the outside.

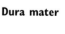

■ Dura mater

■ Arachnoid

■ Pia mater

The meninges are protective membranes forming three distinct layers wrapped right around the brain and spinal cord. In meningitis, these membranes become inflamed through infection.

The dura mater, *the outermost membrane layer, is made from very tough, fibrous material and binds tightly to the inside of the skull.*

The arachnoid membrane *is so called because it looks like a spidery web of criss-crossing fibers. It sits sandwiched between the dura and the pia mater.*

The subarachnoid space *is where the CSF flows; it is the space between the arachnoid and the pia membranes.*

Nerve cells demand so much energy that the brain uses up to 20 percent of the body's oxygen and consumes an incredible 60 percent of its glucose supply.

The pia mater, *the innermost membrane layer, is attached directly to the surface of the cerebrum and follows the contours of the brain.*

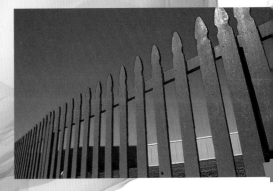

BLOOD–BRAIN BARRIER

Analogous to a "molecular fence," the blood–brain barrier offers another level of protection. To reach the brain, any substance in the bloodstream must traverse a dense network of cells and tightly packed capillaries. These tiny blood vessels present a selective barrier: anything that dissolves in water cannot pass, but fat-soluble substances simply glide across. This defense, however, comes at a price—only certain drugs can reach the brain; anesthetics can whereas most antibiotics cannot. When treating a neurological condition, doctors must be sure that the drug will reach its target within the brain.

Cerebrospinal fluid (CSF)—*a solution of glucose, proteins, vitamins, and other nutrients—bathes the entire nervous system. Together with the blood, this nutrient-rich fluid feeds the energy-hungry nerve cells.*

The neuron

*More than 100 billion nerve cells—known as neurons—
make up the human brain. The building block for the entire
nervous system, these tiny but amazing cells are at the heart
of every brain and body function.*

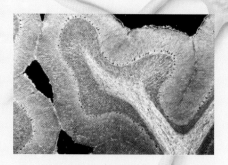

A matter of white and gray
*The brain's gray matter (on the outside) is
made up of the cell bodies of neurons, while
white matter consists of their axons.*

THE BASIC BUILDING BLOCK

Creatures from the humble sea slug to the mighty whale have nervous systems
built from the same basic unit—the nerve cell or neuron. All of the incredible
functions that your brain can perform depend on the abilities of this unique
type of cell, which can stretch hundreds of times the length of the rest of the
cell to make connections with tens of thousands of other neurons. Perhaps the
neuron's most extraordinary quality is that it generates electricity, an energy-
hungry process that gives the brain its amazing capacity for communication,
and explains why it accounts for so much of the body's energy expenditure.

Acting on impulse

Dramatic events within the cell
body generate nerve impulses,
which are passed along the cell's
axon or dendrites, and then
from one neuron to the next.

An axon *is a long projection
that can stretch up to 3.3 feet
to make connections
with other neurons.*

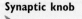

Synaptic knob

Inside the cell *are energy-
making structures and the
nuclear control center.*

The axon hillock
*is the area where
the axon joins the
cell body.*

Dendrites *are
projections from the
main cell body that
make connections with
other neurons and
collect signals from
them. These signals are
passed to the cell body
for "processing."*

The cell body *is the
main part of the neuron
and acts like a computer's
central processor, collecting
inputs from other cells
and determining the
output that is produced.*

Charged particles flood in and
out of the cell, changing the
electrical charge on either side
of the cell membrane. This flux
triggers the same process in the
neighboring part of the axon,
to create a wave of electrical
activity. Such signals are sent
along a series of neurons to
relay information from the brain
to the body. Nerve cells use up a
massive amount of energy as
they pump charged particles in
and out of the cell to prepare
for the next impulse.

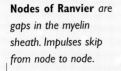

Nodes of Ranvier *are gaps in the myelin sheath. Impulses skip from node to node.*

Synaptic knobs *signify the end of the axon as it branches to connect with other neurons (and with muscle fibers).*

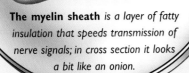

The myelin sheath *is a layer of fatty insulation that speeds transmission of nerve signals; in cross section it looks a bit like an onion.*

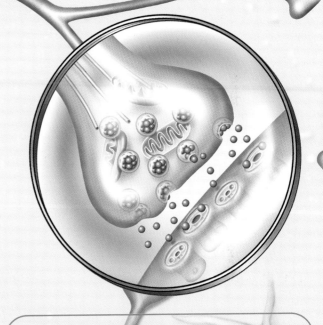

The fast track

Many of the body's neurons are specially adapted for rapid transmission of nerve signals. The axons of these neurons are wrapped in layers of a fatty substance called myelin, a bit like the copper wires of an electrical cable within its rubber insulation. In the brain and spinal cord, myelin sheaths are produced by a type of cell called an oligodendrocyte (elsewhere in the body this function is performed by Schwann cells). Spaced along the length of the myelin sheath are gaps, known as nodes of Ranvier. The nerve signals travel along the axon by jumping between the nodes, skipping the intervening distances.

Bridging the synaptic gap

Where one neuron meets another, it makes a connection via a structure known as a synapse. A typical synapse is where the end of an axon makes contact with another neuron and spreads out to make a little knob. Between the knob and the next neuron there is a tiny space known as the synaptic gap. Nervous signals cross this gap via special chemicals known as neurotransmitters, which are released by the first neuron. They stream across the space, and on arrival at the other side, they trigger the second neuron to generate its own electrical impulse, which travels down its axon until the next synapse, and so on. Neurotransmitters are vital in regulating and directing the function of the brain.

Impulses can travel along nerve fibers at speeds of up to 270 miles per hour.

The neuron and its world

Neurons may be the stars of the show, but they rely on a variety of other cell types—called glial cells—to support their performance. A well-functioning central nervous system demands a cooperative effort from all involved.

TEAM PLAYERS

The central nervous system is made up from a complex web of interconnected cells, supporting, feeding, and communicating with one another. First, there are many different types of neuron, each suited to its particular task. Second, the neurons depend on a supporting cast, the glial cells, to feed them, to protect them from hostile substances or organisms, and to guide their attempts to make contact with one another.

If the cell body of a single neuron were enlarged to the size of a tennis ball, the axon would be well over half a mile long.

LEAN ON ME

Glial cells form a sort of neuron support crew, and incredible though it may seem, they outnumber the latter by up to 50 to 1; there are between 1000 and 5000 billion glial cells in your brain. The name derives from the Greek for glue, which is apt as glial cells bind the brain together. There are several different types—the star-shaped astrocyte, for instance, is one of the most common. They provide structural support, they deliver nutrients to the hungry neurons and clear away their waste products, and they help to intercept toxic substances or dangerous organisms, such as bacteria and viruses. When neurons send out their dendrites in search of other neurons to contact, glial cells help to guide them.

Cast of characters

The nervous system is made up of several different types of neuron; even within the brain there are many different types.

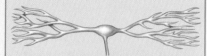

Reticular neurons *are found in the brainstem. They have an axon that splits in two as soon as it leaves the cell body, and then branches many times.*

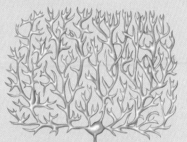

Purkinje cells *are found in the cerebellum. They have a distinctive appearance, with one long axon and an enormously intricate "dendritic tree"— the branching arrangement of dendrites.*

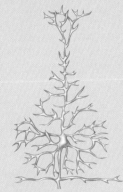

Pyramidal cells *are found in the outer layer of the brain—the cortex—in the area that initiates voluntary muscle movements. They have cell bodies shaped like a pyramid and very long axons that extend all the way down to the brainstem and beyond.*

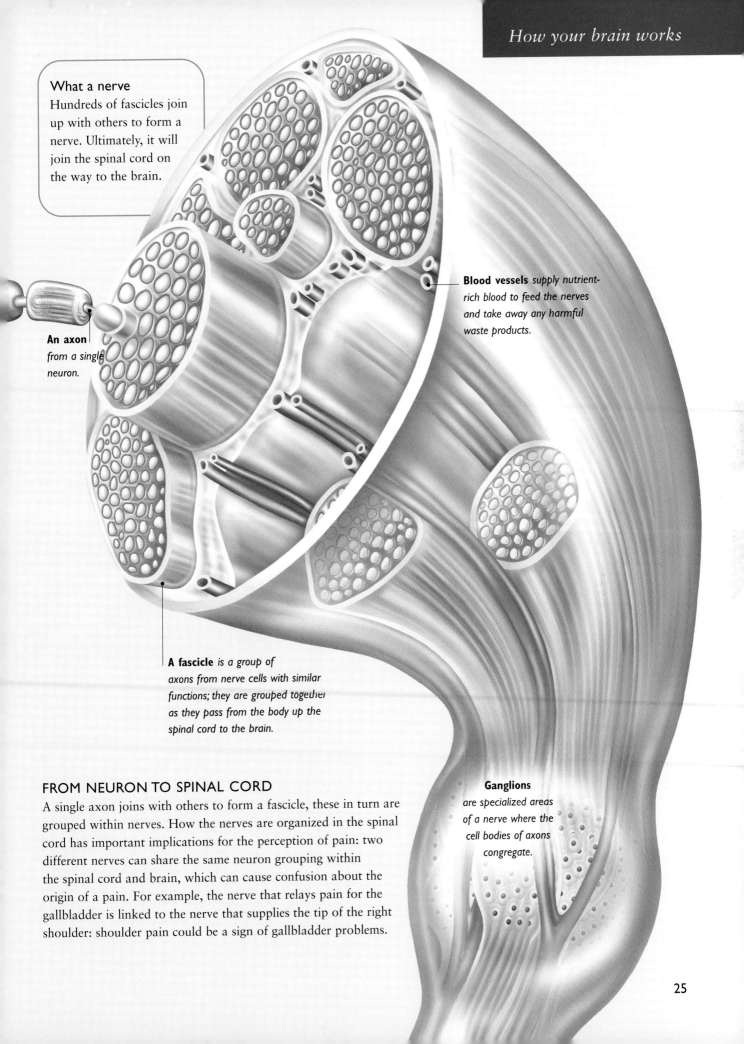

What a nerve
Hundreds of fascicles join up with others to form a nerve. Ultimately, it will join the spinal cord on the way to the brain.

An axon *from a single neuron.*

Blood vessels *supply nutrient-rich blood to feed the nerves and take away any harmful waste products.*

A fascicle *is a group of axons from nerve cells with similar functions; they are grouped together as they pass from the body up the spinal cord to the brain.*

FROM NEURON TO SPINAL CORD
A single axon joins with others to form a fascicle, these in turn are grouped within nerves. How the nerves are organized in the spinal cord has important implications for the perception of pain: two different nerves can share the same neuron grouping within the spinal cord and brain, which can cause confusion about the origin of a pain. For example, the nerve that relays pain for the gallbladder is linked to the nerve that supplies the tip of the right shoulder: shoulder pain could be a sign of gallbladder problems.

Ganglions *are specialized areas of a nerve where the cell bodies of axons congregate.*

The spinal cord

Acting as your own information superhighway, the spinal cord is a vital connection between brain and body. Nerve signals from every single cell feed into it, and orders from the brain are sent out through it.

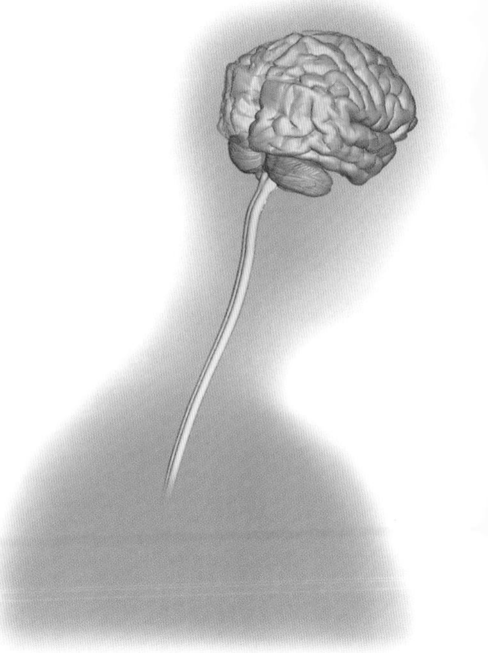

THE LONG BRAIN

In many ways the spinal cord is an extension of the brain. It is constructed of the same white and gray matter as the brain (see page 22), except that in the spine the "pattern" is reversed, with the white matter (axons) surrounding a core of gray matter (neuron cell bodies). In an average adult, the spinal cord extends about 18 in (45 cm) down the back. It terminates between the top two lumbar vertebrae (L1 and L2), just below the waist, which is why doctors can take a sample of cerebrospinal fluid via a procedure called a spinal tap without risk of damage (see page 103). Spinal nerves do run below this level, but they emerge from the cord higher up and then travel down the torso.

The spinal cord carries messages from the brain to the body and relays nerve signals from the body to the brain. However, it is not just a biological telephone cable. Basic processing of nerve signals takes place in the spinal gray matter resulting, for instance, in simple reflex movement.

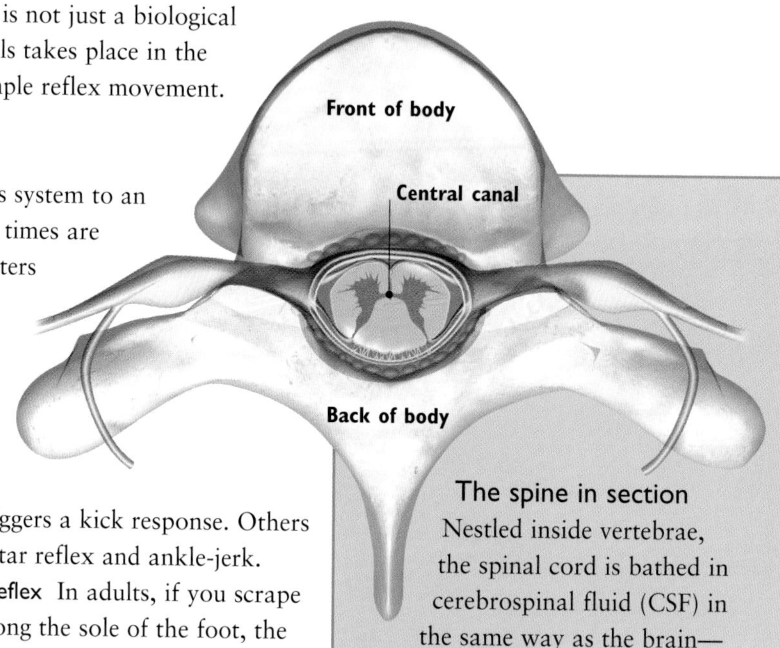

Reflex actions

A reflex is an automatic response of the nervous system to an outside stimulus. In spinal reflexes the response times are incredibly fast: a signal from a sensory nerve enters the spine and instantly triggers a signal in a motor nerve. Spinal reflexes allow you to react much faster than if you had to think about it.

A well-known spinal reflex is the knee-jerk— tapping the leg just below the knee triggers a kick response. Others include the plantar reflex and ankle-jerk.

- **The plantar reflex** In adults, if you scrape something along the sole of the foot, the toes curl under. This reflex is the opposite of the short-lived Babinski reflex in babies in which the toes splay outward.
- **The ankle-jerk reflex** If you tap the tendon just behind the ankle the foot jerks downward.

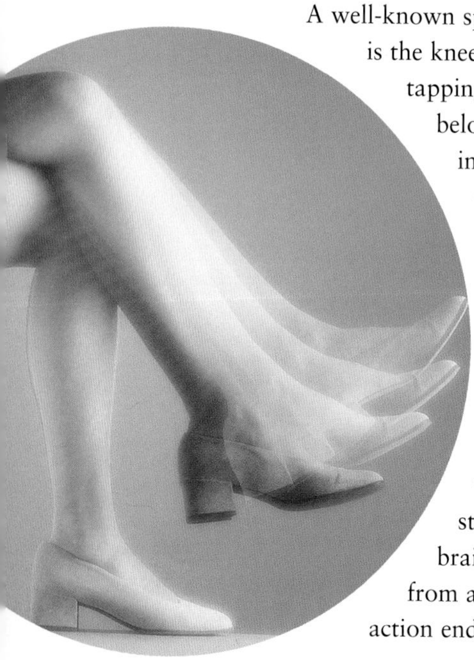

Other reflex actions are not so straightforward and involve input from your brain. For example, withdrawing your hand from a hot object is a reflex reaction, but if this action endangered someone you could override it.

Front of body

Central canal

Back of body

The spine in section
Nestled inside vertebrae, the spinal cord is bathed in cerebrospinal fluid (CSF) in the same way as the brain— it runs between the arachnoid and the pia mater membranes. CSF also circulates in the central canal, which connects to the ventricles in the brain.

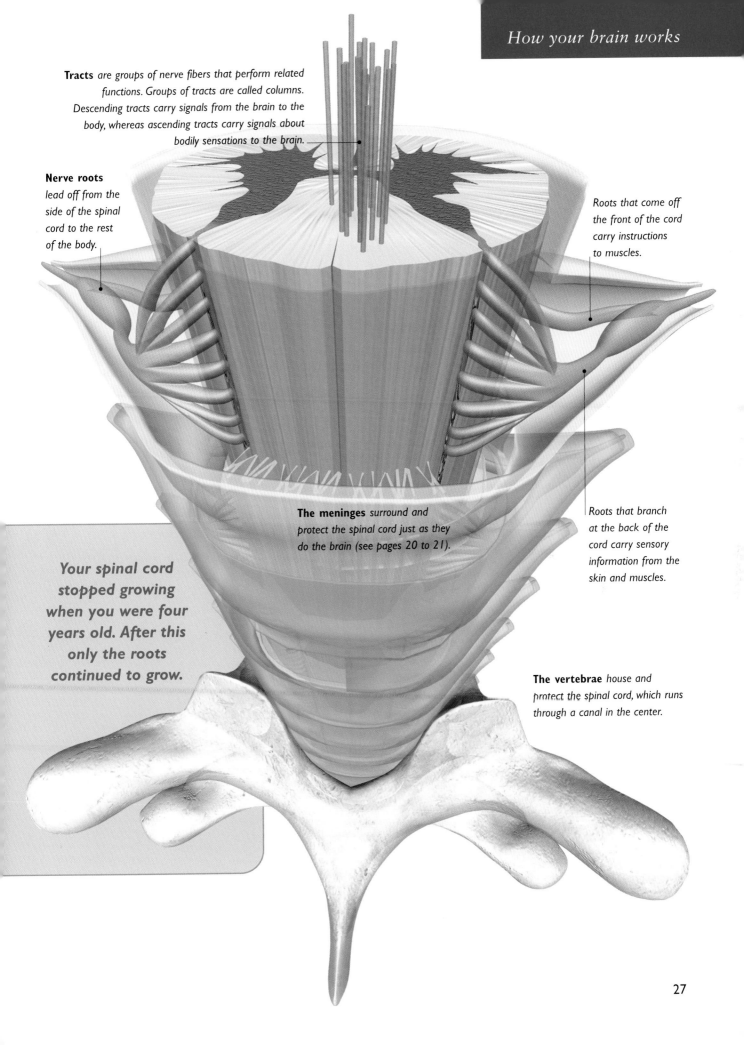

Tracts *are groups of nerve fibers that perform related functions. Groups of tracts are called columns. Descending tracts carry signals from the brain to the body, whereas ascending tracts carry signals about bodily sensations to the brain.*

Nerve roots *lead off from the side of the spinal cord to the rest of the body.*

Roots that come off the front of the cord carry instructions to muscles.

The meninges *surround and protect the spinal cord just as they do the brain (see pages 20 to 21).*

Roots that branch at the back of the cord carry sensory information from the skin and muscles.

Your spinal cord stopped growing when you were four years old. After this only the roots continued to grow.

The vertebrae *house and protect the spinal cord, which runs through a canal in the center.*

Basic divisions of the brain

In anatomical terms, the brain can be subdivided into the three distinct structures of the brainstem, cerebellum, and cerebrum. Separate and yet interdependent, they combine to produce an amazing range of abilities.

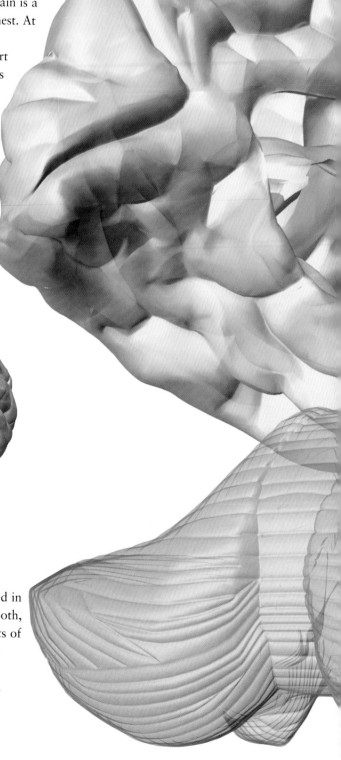

A JOURNEY THROUGH THE BRAIN

Traveling from the spinal cord to the outermost layers of the brain is a journey from the lowest levels of mental functioning to the highest. At the base of the brain is the brainstem—a set of structures that regulates many of the unconscious processes of life, such as heart rate. At the back of the brainstem is the cerebellum, which helps to coordinate both conscious and unconscious elements of movement. Moving on to the large outer portion of the brain—the cerebrum—we find that processing becomes more complex and consciously controlled, allowing us to control our actions and respond to the world around us.

The basics of brain anatomy
Where the spinal cord meets the base of the brain, it swells to give the brainstem. Attached to this is the heavily wrinkled cerebellum. Above them, the grooved surface of the cerebrum makes up most of the visible surface of the brain.

The cerebrum

The cerebellum

The brainstem

The cerebellum

Looking a bit like a brain in miniature, the cerebellum is involved in producing the complex pattern of nerve signals required for smooth, coordinated, and balanced movements. You control many aspects of motion unconsciously, mainly thanks to your cerebellum. This is also where the "programs" for learned movement patterns are coordinated, for instance, the sequence of moves in a golf swing.

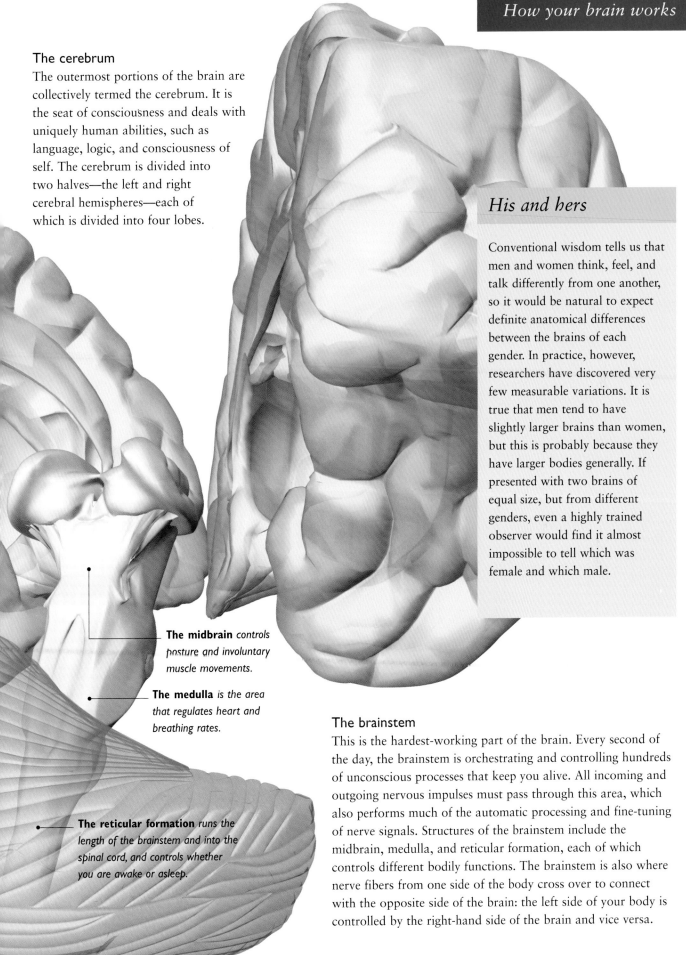

The cerebrum

The outermost portions of the brain are collectively termed the cerebrum. It is the seat of consciousness and deals with uniquely human abilities, such as language, logic, and consciousness of self. The cerebrum is divided into two halves—the left and right cerebral hemispheres—each of which is divided into four lobes.

His and hers

Conventional wisdom tells us that men and women think, feel, and talk differently from one another, so it would be natural to expect definite anatomical differences between the brains of each gender. In practice, however, researchers have discovered very few measurable variations. It is true that men tend to have slightly larger brains than women, but this is probably because they have larger bodies generally. If presented with two brains of equal size, but from different genders, even a highly trained observer would find it almost impossible to tell which was female and which male.

The midbrain *controls posture and involuntary muscle movements.*

The medulla *is the area that regulates heart and breathing rates.*

The reticular formation *runs the length of the brainstem and into the spinal cord, and controls whether you are awake or asleep.*

The brainstem

This is the hardest-working part of the brain. Every second of the day, the brainstem is orchestrating and controlling hundreds of unconscious processes that keep you alive. All incoming and outgoing nervous impulses must pass through this area, which also performs much of the automatic processing and fine-tuning of nerve signals. Structures of the brainstem include the midbrain, medulla, and reticular formation, each of which controls different bodily functions. The brainstem is also where nerve fibers from one side of the body cross over to connect with the opposite side of the brain: the left side of your body is controlled by the right-hand side of the brain and vice versa.

Structures deep within the brain

The thalamus, the hypothalamus, and the structures of the limbic system are among the least understood of the brain's many components, yet they influence your deepest urges and most basic instincts.

THE BRAIN'S PRIMITIVE "HEART"

Between the brainstem and the cerebrum are the limbic system, thalamus, and hypothalamus. These structures provide a link between the unconscious processes performed by the brainstem and the conscious activities of the cerebrum. They are involved in the more "primitive" aspects of being human—emotions, fear, and basic survival drives. They also play essential roles in more "sophisticated" mental abilities, such as learning and memory.

The thalamus and hypothalamus

Information from your senses floods into the thalamus, which sits on top of the brainstem, filtering important and relevant information to the cerebrum. It helps to turn conscious decisions into reality. The hypothalamus is a very small area of tissue with a large area of responsibility. As well as helping to control automatic body processes, such as digestion and urine production, it generates basic drives like hunger, thirst, and even sexual desire. Through its connection with the pituitary gland it controls the secretion of vital hormones.

The limbic system

Most of the brain can be divided into structural groups. The limbic system, however, is a functional group; it includes various structures from different areas of the brain that are involved in functions such as emotion, memory, and learning. Different combinations of the structures perform slightly different functions. For instance, imagine you are walking home one night and encounter a fierce dog. Your amygdala, an almond-shaped structure next to your hypothalamus, helps to produce feelings of fear and apprehension. It also works in conjunction with your hippocampus to link the memory of your canine encounter with the emotions you felt at the time. Your hippocampus works with the mamillary bodies, structures in the base of the hypothalamus, to store these memories, and it is also involved when you are learning a new route home that avoids the dog.

A view from the side
The right cerebral hemisphere has been removed to expose the limbic system in this view.

The fornix *is a tract of white matter that connects the hippocampus with the hypothalamus.*

The thalamus *is the brain's information processing and integrating center; it relays data to higher structures as appropriate.*

The hippocampus, *named for its supposed resemblance to a seahorse, is involved in memory, learning new skills, and recognition.*

The parahippocampal gyrus *sits beneath the hippocampus and helps you to modify expression of feelings.*

A view from behind
This perspective of the structures of the limbic system without the cingulate gyrus clearly shows the two "sides" that sit within each cerebral hemisphere.

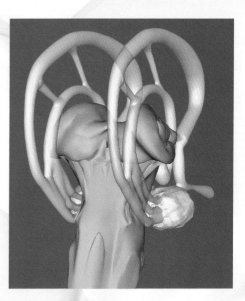

The septum pellucidum *connects the fornix to the bridge between the two cerebral hemispheres—the corpus callosum.*

The cingulate gyrus *is actually a portion of the cerebrum; scientists know that it's part of the limbic system, but its exact functions are unclear.*

The hypothalamus *is a peanut-sized structure that links the brain with the body's hormone system.*

The mamillary body *is a small mass of gray matter in the base of the hypothalamus. It relays information between the fornix and thalamus.*

The amygdala *is involved in emotional expression, aggressive behavior, and processing emotional memories.*

The olfactory bulb *relays information about smells to the limbic system, which helps to explain why a particular scent can evoke powerful memories.*

Higher structures of the brain

The abilities that make us human originate in the outermost layers of the brain—the cerebrum, and in particular its surface, the cerebral cortex. This is where thought, language, logic, and imagination take place.

A BRAIN OF TWO HALVES

One look at the human brain confirms the dominance of the cerebrum—the outer portion of the brain. Its outside surface has two obvious features. One is that it is extremely wrinkled, which allows a lot of brain to be packed into a small space and maximizes the surface area—the most active parts of the cerebrum are in this surface layer, known as the cerebral cortex. The other is that the cerebrum is split into two halves—the cerebral hemispheres. Although visually almost identical, the two hemispheres have different functions. They play profoundly different roles in a number of areas: emotion, language, mathematics, and the way they deal with information from the senses. You are not normally aware of these differences because the two halves are connected by the corpus callosum—a bridge that continuously transfers information back and forth between the two at such high speed that they seem to operate as one. Each hemisphere is made up of four lobes.

Where mind meets matter

The cerebrum is divided into white and gray matter. Its outer surface, known as the cortex, is composed of gray matter—the bodies of nerve cells. Each of these cells is connected to thousands of others in the cortex, allowing an enormous amount of information processing to be carried out. This thin region on the surface of the brain is where all the higher mental functions, such as thought and planning, take place. Beneath the thin layer of gray matter, the greater proportion of the cerebrum is made up of white matter—the long, insulated connecting wires between nerve cells, which link the cortex to all the other parts of the brain.

A one-sided view of life

Because of the way the brain divides its functions between the two cerebral hemispheres, damage to one can produce an unusual condition called unilateral neglect. Affected people unconsciously ignore one side of space, with bizarre consequences such as:

- shaving only one side of the face;
- putting all the numbers in one half when asked to draw a clock;
- eating only the food on one side of the plate, even though they may still be hungry;
- not recognizing limbs on the "wrong" side of the body: a sufferer may even attempt to throw a "stranger's leg" out of bed.

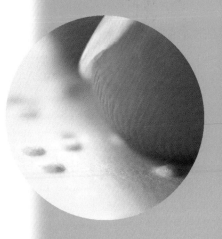

The parietal lobes
Located at the back and top of the brain, the parietal lobes contain the area where sensations from different parts of the body are consciously felt.

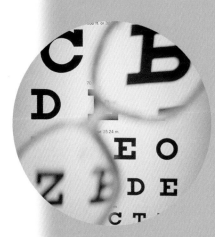

The occipital lobes
These sit at the back of the brain and are mainly concerned with vision.

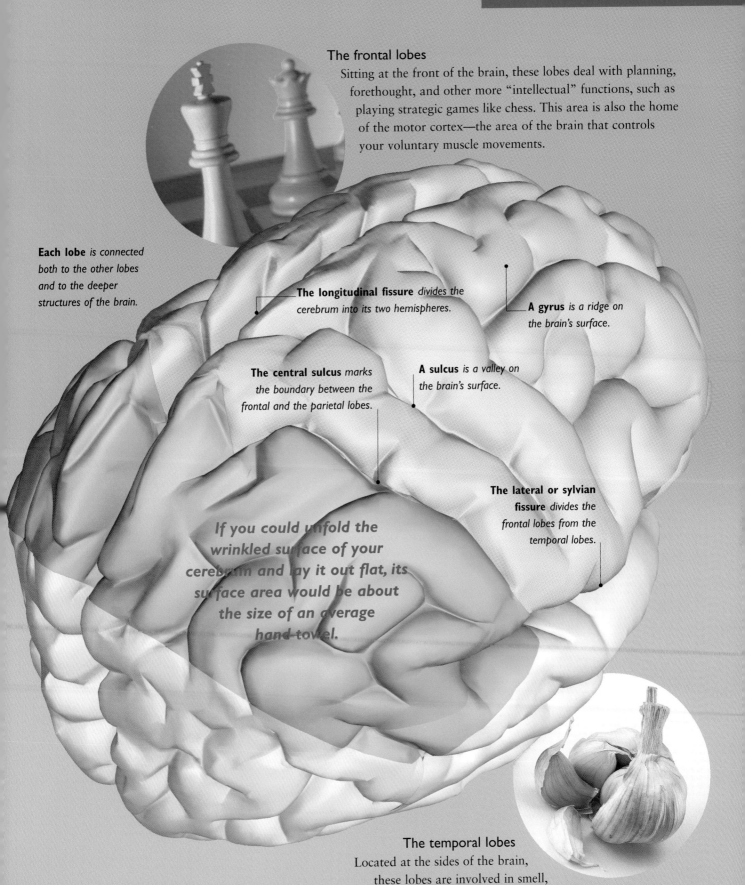

The frontal lobes
Sitting at the front of the brain, these lobes deal with planning, forethought, and other more "intellectual" functions, such as playing strategic games like chess. This area is also the home of the motor cortex—the area of the brain that controls your voluntary muscle movements.

Each lobe *is connected both to the other lobes and to the deeper structures of the brain.*

The longitudinal fissure *divides the cerebrum into its two hemispheres.*

A gyrus *is a ridge on the brain's surface.*

The central sulcus *marks the boundary between the frontal and the parietal lobes.*

A sulcus *is a valley on the brain's surface.*

The lateral or sylvian fissure *divides the frontal lobes from the temporal lobes.*

If you could unfold the wrinkled surface of your cerebrum and lay it out flat, its surface area would be about the size of an average hand towel.

The temporal lobes
Located at the sides of the brain, these lobes are involved in smell, hearing, and making sense of language.

Mapping brain functions

One of the most exciting fields of brain research is the attempt to map the activities of the brain, in particular to pinpoint which part of the outer layer of the brain—the cerebral cortex—performs which higher brain function.

The left hemisphere *is dominant for brain activity related to logic, math, and language.*

WHAT HAPPENS WHERE?

Despite extensive research, scientists have found that function can rarely be isolated to one specific site in the cerebral cortex; many different parts of the brain can be involved in a mental activity, and there are no clear borders between areas. Nonetheless, we can roughly map where the cortex deals with mental functions. Such a map clearly demonstrates the left–right division of higher functions such as language processing and spatial reasoning.

PICKING, MATCHING, AND MIXING

All of the body's senses—sight, hearing, smell, taste, and touch—are linked to their own region of the cortex. The organization of this outer layer of the brain can be broken down into three broad zones of function.

- **Picking out detail** Raw information from the senses is dealt with by "primary cortical areas." In the primary visual cortex, for instance, sets of neurons fire in response to different lines: horizontal, vertical, curved, etc. When you see a person's face, various neurons respond to the lines that make up the face.

- **Matching to make a whole** Next to the primary cortex are the "associative areas," which link different types of information. For example, horizontal lines constitute one type of information, diagonal ones another. The visual associative cortex puts them together, allowing you to recognize a complex collection of lines as a face.

- **Mixing with other kinds of information** The next stage of processing is performed by the "integrative areas." These attach meaning to things you recognize and perform complicated functions, such as predicting the outcome of a course of action. The visual integrative area, for example, links the face with the name of the person it belongs to.

b

c

Learning about function—Gage's brain

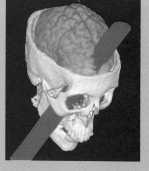

In the past, brain function was studied by seeing what happens when part of the brain is damaged. A famous case was that of Phineas Gage. In 1848, an industrial accident near Cavendish, Vermont, blew a long metal rod through the front of his brain. To everyone's amazement, he recovered physically, but his personality changed overnight: He went from being considerate and responsible to being foul mouthed, bad tempered, and incapable of making any long-term plans. In 1994 a computer reconstruction showed that Gage had suffered damage to precisely the area now believed to control rational behavior and forethought.

The right hemisphere
*is dominant for brain activity
related to emotions and art.*

A key to brain function

a **Associative and primary
motor cortex** are the parts of the
brain that work together to produce
writing movements.

b **The left auditory cortex**
analyzes signals from the right ear.

c **The general interpretive
center** or **Wernicke's area** allows
words to be combined to give
meaning to sentences and performs
your mathematical calculations.

d **The right visual cortex** is
where information from the left-hand
side of space (as opposed to just the
left eye) is analyzed. When you
watch TV, each eye sees both sides of
the screen, but only things happening
on the left of the screen are "seen"
by this side of the brain.

e **The spatial integrative area**
processes information related to
where things are in space.

f **The associative and primary
sensory cortex** work together to
tell you what object you are holding
by touch.

g **The prefrontal cortex** is
involved in a range of functions,
including planning and forethought.

Sensation and motion

Humans are capable of an enormous range of sensations and movements because our brains have evolved a number of highly complex structures, from the cerebellum to the cerebral cortex.

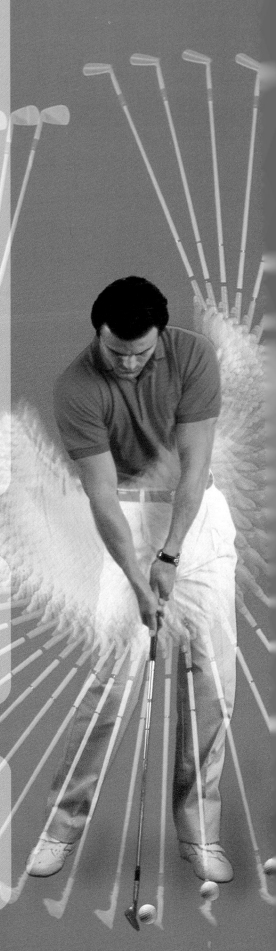

STRIP FOR SUCCESS

Running down either side of the central sulcus (the trench that divides the frontal from the parietal lobes) are two strips of cortex that allow you to sense your skin and muscles, and to move your limbs. To the front of the sulcus is the motor (muscle-controlling) strip, and to the rear is the somatosensory (body-sensing) strip. In a normal person, these two narrow strips of tissue, each just 3/16 inch thick, are capable of producing a huge range of movement and sensation, from sweeps of the arm to tiny twitches of the fingers and from heat to the lightest pressure of a pinprick. Damage to either or both of these strips, for instance as a result of a stroke, can result in paralysis and/or loss of sensation.

EASY AS 1-2-3

Many movements, such as a golf swing, combine conscious and unconscious brain processes. Here we follow these processes to see how the brain combines them to control the movements of a golf drive.

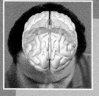

1 The ball is on the tee and the club is in your hand. Information from the muscles of your arm is relayed via the brainstem and thalamus to the somatosensory strip, giving you the conscious sensation of weight. The neighboring parietal lobe then gets involved, helping you to understand what the 'weight' signals mean. Now the frontal lobe is called into play to decide how far away the hole is and how hard you need to hit the ball.

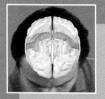

2 Your frontal lobes have made a decision about how you need to hit the ball. The parts of the frontal lobe next to the motor strip plan out the necessary sequence of moves to produce the required swing. In just milliseconds the plan is in place and the nerve cells in the parts of the motor strip that correspond to the relevant muscles fire. Signals are sent to these muscles via the brainstem and spinal cord.

In humans, the most represented areas in the somatosensory cortex are the fingers, lips, and tongue. But in the somatosensory cortex of a rabbit, the nose commands the most space.

Somatosensory strip

Motor strip

Central sulcus

Premotor and supplementary motor areas *are active when you think about performing a movement, before you actually carry it out.*

The somatosensory and motor strips
These areas of cortex run down either side of the central sulcus. Each strip has a neighboring area that is involved in determining what sensations mean and in planning the movements you intend to make.

Homunculus

Scientists studying the motor and somatosensory strips have discovered that the body is represented on the surface of the cortex like a map. At one end of the motor strip, for example, the muscles of the toes and feet are represented, and the next portion relates to the nerve cells for the leg, and so on, up to the face and mouth. Not all body parts are represented equally. The trunk of the body commands relatively little space, whereas the hands, feet, and lips map a lot of area. Below, the "homunculus" (little man) shows the proportions of these features relating to their representation on the motor strip.

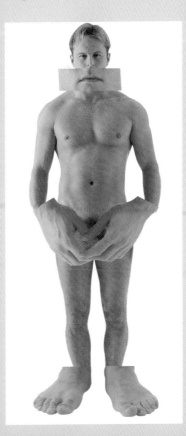

3 Meanwhile, your basal ganglia—masses of gray matter buried deep in the cerebrum—are also active, controlling fine details such as balancing the rest of your body so that you don't fall over. Fine-tuning of coordination is further helped by the cerebellum. For instance, while you are concentrating on your trunk and arms, your leg and back muscles have to adjust and maintain their tone to help you remain steady and upright—which is where the cerebellum comes in.

Memory

You possess an extraordinary capacity for storing information—from names and dates to complex skills—the limits of which are rarely fully stretched and still only poorly understood.

MEMORY LANE

Many people in their '80s or '90s can vividly remember tiny details from childhood events. How are these mental feats possible, particularly when many of us often cannot remember where we put something only hours or even minutes before?

It is now known that memory operates in three stages—sensory, short-term and long-term. The first stage, sensory memory, lasts for between 0.25 and 3 seconds; signals from your senses rattle around your brain and unless they attract your attention for some reason, they will simply disappear. Important information proceeds to stage two, short-term memory, where it remains for about 30 seconds. Particularly significant data is then transferred to long-term memory—stage three—where it can be stored for anything from a few hours to a lifetime. Memories become stored permanently with repeated practice and use.

What does a memory look like?

Is it possible to put a slice of brain under the microscope and point to a structure that represents an actual memory? In the 1960s, researchers studied patients undergoing brain surgery (who were conscious) and stimulated areas on the outer surface with tiny electrodes. They found that the same memory could be triggered by stimulating different spots. This suggested that a single memory involves nerve cells in several different areas of the brain, which led to a current theory that memories are encoded in circuits of neurons. One particular pattern of firing in a circuit represents one memory, but another pattern involving the same neurons and circuit triggers a different one.

The cortex, *the outermost layer of the cerebrum, is where long-term memories are stored.*

The hippocampus *is pivotal in laying down long-term memories. If it is missing, as a result of injury or surgery, new skills can still be learned but there will be no recollection of having learned them.*

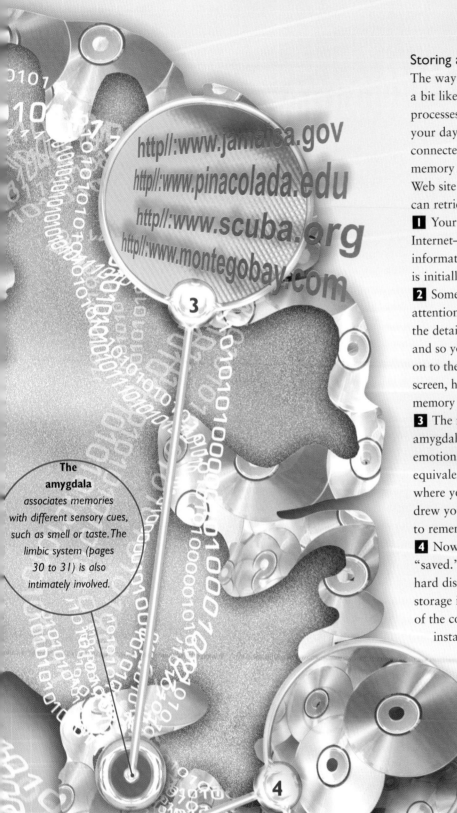

http//:www.jamaica.gov
http//:www.pinacolada.edu
http//:www.scuba.org
http//:www.montegobay.com

3

The amygdala *associates memories with different sensory cues, such as smell or taste. The limbic system (pages 30 to 31) is also intimately involved.*

4

Storing a memory

The way that your brain forms new memories is a bit like the way that a personal computer (PC) processes and stores information. Imagine that your day-to-day life is like being a PC on-line, connected to the Internet. Laying down a memory is like finding some information on a Web site and then saving it on your PC, so you can retrieve it at your leisure.

1 Your senses are like a continuous link to the Internet—they carry a constant flood of information from the outside world, all of which is initially relayed to your brain.

2 Some of this information captures your attention for some reason—perhaps, for example, the details of a vacation you are interested in— and so your brain takes note. This data then moves on to the hippocampus, which acts like a computer screen, holding it in the computer's working memory and displaying it for you to look at.

3 The next stop for the information is the amygdala, which is involved in attaching emotional significance. This is the mental equivalent of noting down the Web site addresses where you found the information or noting what drew you there. These associations will help you to remember the information and retrieve it.

4 Now the information is ready to be stored or "saved." A computer would save it in a file on its hard disk or on a CD. The equivalent permanent storage in your brain is the cortex. Different parts of the cortex store different types of memory. For instance the visual cortex stores visual memories, so pictorial information is stored here, complete with the associations made by the amygdala. When you retrieve your memory of this Web page— perhaps set off by seeing something that reminds you of the picture—you are effectively calling up the file saved on your cortex.

Language

Neuroscientists generally regard language as the most quintessentially human ability. The ability to speak coherently and to understand language depends on the complex interaction of speech centers in the brain, which coordinate the subtleties of meaning, vocabulary, and articulation.

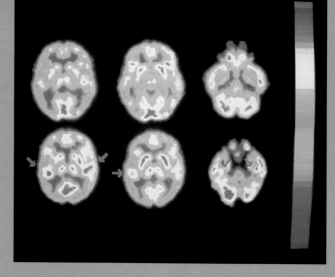

The activity of listening
These brain scans show brain activity (low in blue, high in red) of different brain areas. To determine the many parts involved in listening to words, researchers compared the patterns of someone sitting quietly (top row) with those of the same person undertaking a simple listening exercise. The shift in the pattern of red is clearly visible.

LANGUAGE IN MIND

Many philosophers argue that language is central to consciousness and a vital part of what makes us human. Naturally, therefore, a lot of attention has been paid to how language is produced and understood by the brain. From the landmark discoveries of the 19th century, up to the present day, psychologists and doctors have investigated language function and dysfunction to try to find the answers to these questions.

> **Ninety-six percent of right-handed people and 70 percent of left-handed people are left-brain-hemisphere dominant for language; 15 percent of left-handed people have mixed dominance, with language abilities shared between both hemispheres.**

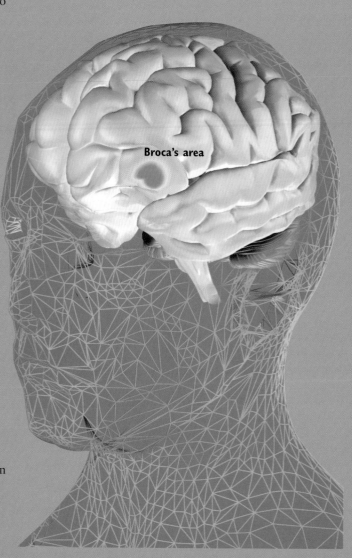

Broca's area

Broca's area—putting words in your mouth
One of the vital language areas in the brain is part of the left frontal lobe, known as Broca's area. It is named after a 19th-century French physician who linked brain damage to this specific area with a specific language problem. People who had suffered such damage could understand language and had normal intelligence, but were unable to form coherent speech beyond the odd word or noise (a condition known as Broca's aphasia). Broca, therefore, deduced that this was the part of the brain that produced the complex sequence of movements used in speaking.

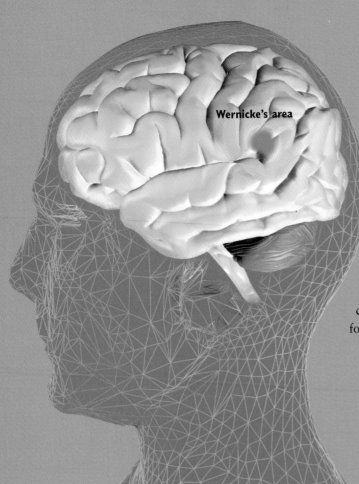

Wernicke's area

Wernicke's area—meaning what you say

Also vital for speech is a region of the left temporal lobe known as Wernicke's area. This is named after a researcher who discovered that patients with damage to this part of the brain produced fluent-sounding speech that lacked any meaning (a condition known as Wernicke's aphasia). Such patients produce a rapid stream of speech with all the usual rhythms and intonations, but composed of words and nonsense syllables in a mix described as "word salad." They also had trouble comprehending what was said to them. Wernicke concluded that this part of the brain must be responsible for understanding and producing meaning in language.

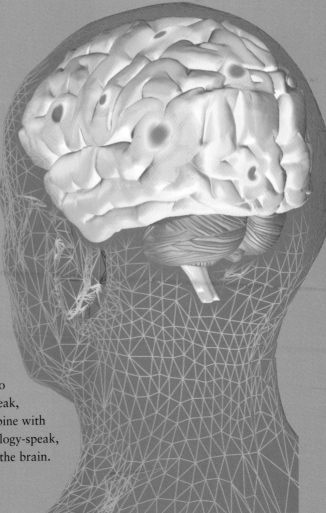

Making sense of it all

Early models of language in the brain pictured the content of speech being produced by Wernicke's area and then passed on to Broca's area to be turned into the mouth, tongue, and vocal cord movements needed. Recent research, however, suggests that many other parts of the cortex are also involved. When you hear someone speak, the sounds are processed by several areas at once, including Wernicke's, and they combine to build up a conscious understanding of language. When you speak, something similar happens—several different regions combine with Broca's area to convert your thoughts into sounds. In psychology-speak, language abilities are "distributed" around the brain.

How the brain controls the body

Your brain and spinal cord work in partnership with your body's peripheral nervous system. This network of nerves not only feeds information to your brain but controls a whole host of conscious and unconscious body functions.

THE NERVOUS SYSTEM NETWORK

The brain and spinal cord make up the central nervous system. The rest of the body is served by the peripheral nervous system, a network of nerves that feeds into the spine, relaying signals between the brain and the muscles, skin, and organs of the body. Together these two systems make up the body's nervous system. They are in constant communication, controlling every movement and action—both conscious and unconscious.

The peripheral nervous system breaks down into two subdivisions. One set—the somatic system of nerves—sends sensory information to your brain and also connects to the muscles that you can consciously control. Another set—the autonomic system— connects to the parts of the body that operate unconsciously, such as your heart and the muscles of your stomach and intestines. The autonomic network itself has two subdivisions—the sympathetic and parasympathetic systems (see below). The whole system is summarized in the diagram on the right.

NERVOUS SYSTEM

PERIPHERAL NERVOUS SYSTEM	CENTRAL NERVOUS SYSTEM
Spinal and cranial nerves	Brain and spinal cord

SOMATIC SYSTEM	AUTONOMIC SYSTEM
Relays messages from the central nervous system to voluntary muscles	Regulates the function of involuntary muscles and glands

SYMPATHETIC SYSTEM	PARASYMPATHETIC SYSTEM
Prepares the body for activity and use of energy	Relaxes the body for the restoration of energy

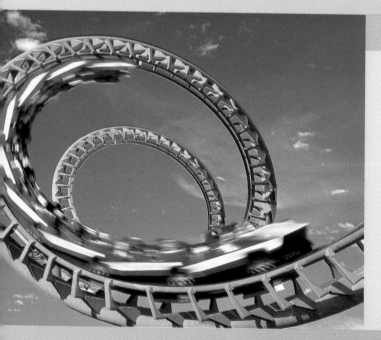

Sympathetic versus parasympathetic

The two branches of the autonomic system work in opposing harmony to balance each other's actions.

- **The sympathetic nervous system** This network initiates the fight-or-flight response in times of stress or danger. Someone getting in line for an amusement park ride, for example, may well be feeling nervous, which swings the sympathetic nerves into action, resulting in a dry mouth, dilated pupils, sweaty skin, and a racing heart.
- **The parasympathetic nervous system** Once the rollercoaster ride is over, the "passenger" relaxes and the parasympathetic network takes control to return the body to normal: sweating stops; the pupils constrict; the heartbeat slows, along with the breathing rate; and saliva is again secreted to rehydrate the dry mouth.

The central nervous system
consists of the brain and spinal cord.

Cranial nerves *exist as 12 pairs,
which arise from the underside of the
brain. Mostly, they supply the head, face,
neck, and shoulders.*

Spinal nerves *exit the spinal
cord in pairs and then divide to
supply the whole body.*

**The autonomic
nervous system** *controls
involuntary body functions
to maintain a constant
internal environment. For
example, it regulates blood
pressure and body
temperature.*

The somatic nervous system
*controls your conscious movements.
When you want to wiggle your big toe,
this system works in conjunction with
your brain and spinal cord to turn
your wish into a reality.*

Parasympathetic nerves *arise
at the top (cranial) and bottom (sacral)
of the nervous system. They act on the
optic nerve, for example, to dilate the
pupil and also on the facial nerve, which
controls salivary and tear gland
secretions.*

**The sympathetic nervous
system** *arises from the spinal cord and
forms a line of ganglia (clusters of
neuron cell bodies) that run alongside.
This set of nerves influences gut function
during digestion and regulates body
temperature.*

A day in the life of the brain

*If your brain controls your body, what controls your brain?
Both its own chemicals—neurotransmitters—and hormones
regulate your brain's activity, and it follows a number of
cycles that are set by its own internal "clock."*

A CHEMICAL WORLD

Every minute of the day your brain is bathed in a soup of chemicals—
hormones and message-signaling chemicals called neurotransmitters. Many
of these never spread farther than a few thousandths of a millimeter from
where they are released and have very specific effects—for instance, making
a neighboring nerve cell fire off a signal. Others are carried to every corner of
your brain, producing a variety of long-lasting, far-reaching effects. By
influencing these chemicals your body is able to influence your brain,
providing the driving force behind many of the things you do and feel.

7:30 A.M. Waking up

Even without an alarm, your body knows
roughly when to wake you up. You have an
internal body clock, but where is this clock?
Scientists have pinned it down to a neuron
cluster called the suprachiasmatic nucleus,
which gets extra assistance from the pineal
gland. Located deep within the brainstem,
the pineal gland secretes the sleep-inducing
hormone melatonin and responds to light.
After peaking during the night, increased levels
of melatonin drop off in the morning and your
brain revs up, bringing you to wakefulness.

8:30 A.M. Commuting

The journey to work is often stressful, triggering the
fight-or-flight response that readies your body systems
for action. One consequence of stress is the production
of a hormone called epinephrine, which is released into the
bloodstream and then courses around your body and affects
many organs, including your brain. Here, it increases blood flow
and heightens alertness, helping you to concentrate on the potentially
dangerous and difficult task of negotiating your route to work.

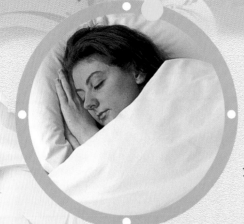

12:30 A.M. And so to sleep

By this time the lack of sunlight triggers your pineal gland to produce high levels of melatonin. Cued by this signal, your suprachiasmatic nucleus sends out signals that shut down the higher portions of your consciousness, sending you to sleep.

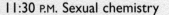

11:30 P.M. Sexual chemistry

When it comes to primitive urges, your brain is at the mercy of body chemicals. Your libido is partly determined by levels of testosterone, whereas hormones such as oxytocin act on the brain to produce everything from intense infatuation to uncontrollable lust. Orgasm is accompanied by the production of a flood of neurotransmitters such as dopamine, which gives sensations of euphoria and well-being.

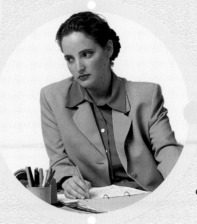

3 P.M. Mid-afternoon slump

You're back at your desk, but increased blood levels of sugars from the food you have eaten cause a rise in the levels of the neurotransmitter serotonin. This acts on your brain to lift your mood, but can also make you drowsy, bringing on a mid-afternoon slump.

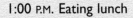

1:00 P.M. Eating lunch

Falling blood levels of glucose prompt the hunger centers of your brain into action, driving you into the cafeteria or snack bar for nourishment. Once you have eaten, a different set of responses takes over—a full stomach triggers the release of a hormone called cholecystokinin, which relays this fact to your brain; so you feel full.

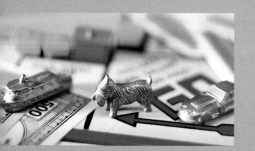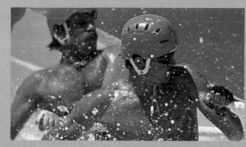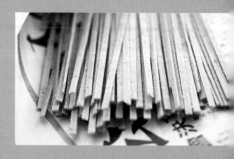

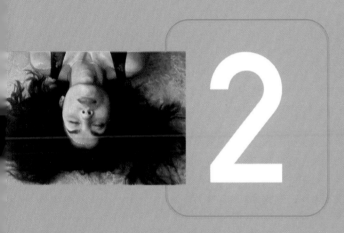

2

Brain-healthy living

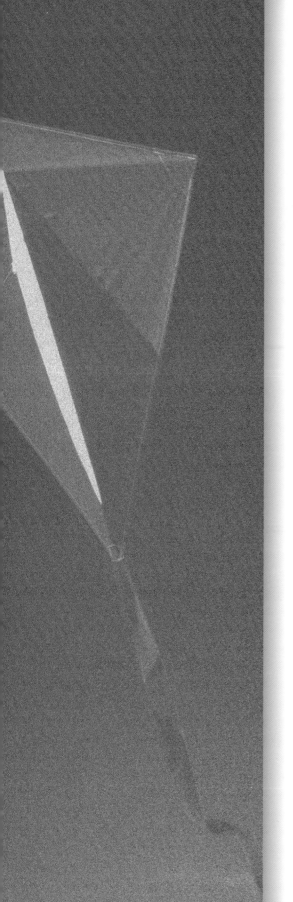

TAKE CHARGE OF YOUR BRAIN HEALTH

How risky is your life in terms of your brain and central nervous system? Taking sensible precautions when you play a favorite sport, for example, is essential for protecting yourself. Being self-aware is also vital; learn which symptoms are cause for concern and should prompt you to take action and visit your doctor. Work with your doctor to keep your brain and body healthy and in the best possible shape. If you look after your heart, your brain will benefit; adopting an anti-stroke lifestyle will guard against disease from within.

Do you know the most common risk factors for brain health? Find out how to protect your brain and which symptoms might be serious.

Protect your heart and prevent stroke—the number three killer in the developed world—by eating right, exercising, and not smoking.

Babies lose some of the reflexes they were born with, which is normal. How do doctors monitor neurological health through life?

The power of the mind should never be underestimated; learn how to tap into it and how to think more positively.

Safeguarding your brain health

The brain is vulnerable to a variety of risks throughout life, from before birth to old age. Some simple measures can help to safeguard and protect it, both from external risks and from factors stemming from within the body.

Your brain and spinal cord are protected by the skull, vertebrae, and cerebrospinal fluid. But there are a number of factors, inside and outside the body, that can put the health of your central nervous system at risk. Internal risk factors include genetic influences, over which you have no control, and disorders affecting other parts of the body—for example, diabetes mellitus and cardiovascular problems. External risk factors include physical impacts and injury, disease-causing organisms, and toxic chemicals.

These risk factors change in their relative importance throughout life, from the womb to old age.

Extra special care
Special care is needed when handling a baby's head. Although a baby's skull offers some protection to the brain, the skull is still soft, and two small holes, the fontanelles, allow for growth.

PREGNANCY AND BIRTH

In the womb, the main risks to the developing brain are from inadequate nutrition and from poisons that may cross the placenta. By maintaining a healthy diet, avoiding drugs, and limiting alcohol intake, a woman can protect her baby's vulnerable brain and nervous system.

Older mothers and parents with a family history of inherited or congenital disorders are most at risk of bearing handicapped children and may be offered screening early in pregnancy. Tests such as amniocentesis can reveal the presence of some disorders.

Averting labor problems

One of the main risks during labor is the interruption of a baby's blood supply—for instance, pressure on the umbilical cord. If the oxygen supply to an infant's brain is stopped, even briefly, it can cause brain damage leading to cerebral palsy. It is important to have skilled professionals on hand during childbirth to guard against this possibility, whether the baby is born in the hospital or at home.

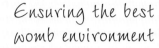

Ensuring the best womb environment

Your baby gets all its nourishment from your bloodstream, via the placenta, so make sure you eat a healthy diet rich in minerals and vitamins. Folate (folic acid) is vital for the development of your baby's brain and nervous system. Folic acid supplements, ideally taken before and during the first three months of pregnancy, reduce the risk of neural tube defects such as spina bifida.

It is also important that the developing brain is protected against hazards. The placenta acts like a barrier, keeping out potentially dangerous molecules, but some substances, such as alcohol, can cross the placenta. For this reason, alcohol intake should be kept well below the usual levels recommended as safe for an adult woman.

Guarding the fontanelles

The bones of the skull have not finished developing at birth and are still soft enough to allow some distortion as the baby squeezes through the birth canal. Although the head quickly resumes a normal shape, two small gaps in the skull, called fontanelles, are left on the top of the head where the bones do not yet meet. The smaller of the two, toward the crown of the head, closes at about six weeks, but the larger opening, nearer to the front of the head, does not disappear until 9 to 18 months. Examining a newborn's

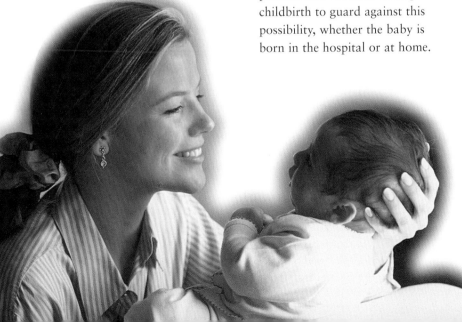

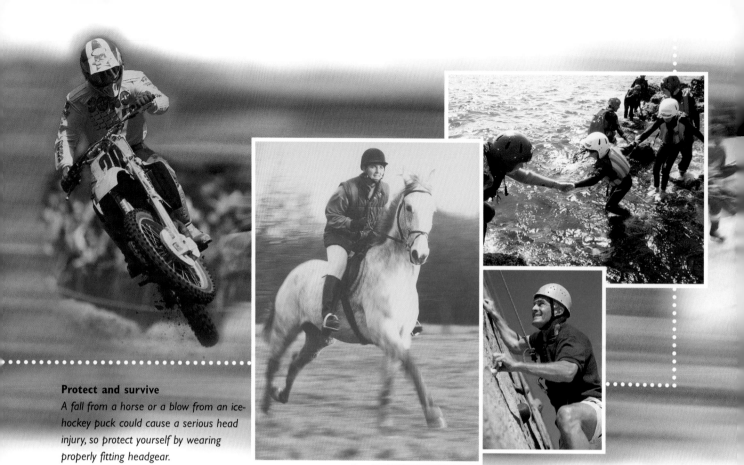

Protect and survive
A fall from a horse or a blow from an ice-hockey puck could cause a serious head injury, so protect yourself by wearing properly fitting headgear.

Is there a risk "thermostat"?

As life gets ever faster and more complex, we rely on experts to make things safer. But studies suggest that in fact we have a risk "thermostat." When a change decreases our perception of risk, our sense of vulnerability is reduced, so we adjust our behavior accordingly. For example, when road engineers straighten a dangerous bend, we simply drive faster.

It could be argued that this is a good thing: journey times by car are decreased, while the risk stays the same for drivers. But higher vehicle speeds can make life harder for others, such as pedestrians and cyclists.

head may reveal a pulsing through the scalp, mirroring the baby's heart beat. This is perfectly normal, but it does mean that everyone should take particular care when handling a baby's head. If the skin over the fontanelle is shrunken or depressed, it can be a sign of dehydration.

CHILDREN AND ADULTS

From infancy through teenage years, the brain grows and matures, reaching its adult form around the age of 20. During these years, and for the next couple of decades, the major risks to the central nervous system come from the outside world—from physical injury or trauma and from infectious organisms. Children and young adults can be at risk from disease organisms, particularly those that cause meningitis. The best defense is to be alert to telltale signs—severe headache and fever, dislike of bright light, and possibly a rash that does

not fade when pressed under a glass—and to have your child immunized.

External risk factors

Until people reach their mid-40s, the major risks to the nervous system are head and spinal injury. The brain and spinal cord are fragile organs, easily damaged by blows to the head or injury to the neck or back. Such trauma is usually the result of automobile accidents. Teaching your children about road safety as pedestrians and ensuring that they cycle, skateboard, or roller skate with proper protection, as well as following safety rules yourself, are the best guarantees of brain safety. Equally, drivers should behave responsibly on the road and pay attention to speed limits, especially in residential areas, and to road and weather conditions.

Participation in sports is another leading cause of brain and spine

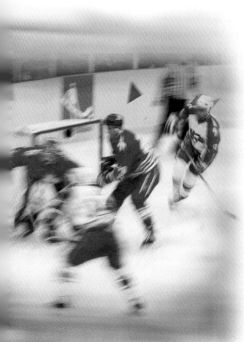

injury, and some sports are riskier than others. Soccer and horseback riding carry the greatest risk of spinal injury; diving into shallow water is a tragically common cause of broken necks and backs.

SPORTS SAFETY

Anyone who participates in sports automatically assumes a certain level of risk. The nature of most sports is to exert the body, putting strain and stress on it and placing it in risk situations. Risk to the brain and spine can be minimized in a number of ways. The most obvious, for sports ranging from ice hockey to automobile racing, is to wear a helmet. Other protective gear includes back protectors for motor-cyclists, harnesses for climbers, and baseball players. Check out the safety equipment for your sport and use it.

In some risky sports, such as soccer and judo, helmets aren't really an option. Head, neck and back safety is best ensured by using the correct technique. The first thing taught in judo, for example, is how to fall safely, by slapping an arm out straight onto the mat to absorb the energy of the impact.

CHANGING RISK FACTORS

As you age, the focus of health risks to your brain and nervous system switches from the outside world back to inside your body. Advancing years increasingly bring the threat of cancer and degenerative diseases, such as Alzheimer's disease, along with a higher risk of heart problems.

The global killer

Stroke is one of the biggest killers in the developed world, so look after your heart health and visit your doctor for advice as necessary. If you have high blood pressure or are receiving treatment for narrowing of the arteries—atherosclerosis— your doctor will already have enrolled you on a program of regular health checks. It will pay health dividends in the future to be well informed about how to prevent or reduce the risk of stroke and how to protect your brain by looking after your heart (see pages 54 to 55).

INCREASE YOUR AWARENESS

Since threats to your brain health can have such serious consequences, it is important to receive treatment as early as possible. Recognizing the significant danger signals could help you get to a doctor in time or allay your fears and anxieties.

Many of the most common neurological symptoms, however, can be vague or generalized—most people have headaches from time to time, for instance. Being over sensitive to the health threat posed by symptoms such as headaches, fatigue, or eyestrain can do more harm than good, and it is important not to worry. Techniques to aid a sensible attitude toward stress are outlined on pages 62 to 65.

Be alert to possible problems

Some disorders of the central nervous system, such as Alzheimer's disease, appear gradually over a period of months or years, so

(see pages 54 to 55).

Are your symptoms serious?

Sometimes it is difficult to know if something is serious or not, especially with symptoms such as headache or tiredness. Think about how you would answer the following questions before you see your doctor.

- *Is the symptom new or is it something you've had before? If you hardly ever get headaches and suddenly experience a blinding pain, it is more likely to be serious.*

- *Has the symptom lasted for more than two weeks? We all feel tired at times, but if you've been exhausted for two weeks, don't ignore it.*

- *Is the symptom getting worse? For instance, if you woke with pins and needles in your arm, it's most likely that you slept on it. But if the sensation worsens rather than lessens, you should see a doctor at once.*

- *Do you have more than one symptom? When two or more symptoms occur together, they may be of more concern.*

HELP YOUR DOCTOR TO HELP YOU

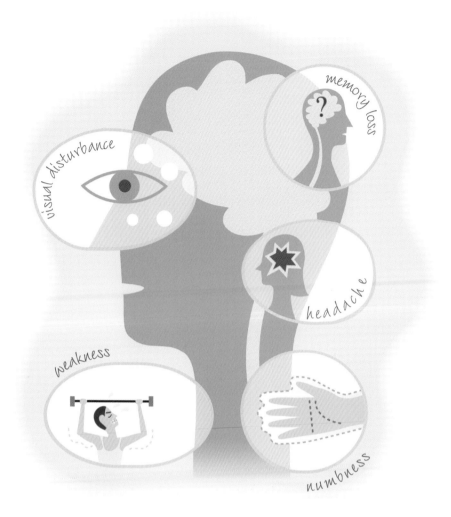

visual disturbance

memory loss

headache

weakness

numbness

Spot the warning signs

Some symptoms can be a warning of a serious condition. Symptoms to be aware of are headache, visual disturbance, memory loss, numbness and physical weakness.

a problem that requires attention may be fairly obvious. Other disorders cause seemingly minor or short-lived symptoms that many people are tempted to ignore. But sometimes, being alert to short-lived symptoms could save your life. For example, temporary blindness could indicate a life-threatening blood clot. Spotting an imminent stroke gives doctors a chance to prescribe vital drugs, whereas knowing the signs of meningitis and acting promptly could save a child's life.

Symptoms to watch

Keeping an eye out for signs and building a store of information by monitoring any change in the nature of symptoms will help your doctor when discussing any problem. Warning signs of a neurological problem include the following.

- **Headache** In the vast majority of cases, headaches are caused by muscle tension, foods, or excess alcohol or sleep. Very rarely an underlying brain or nervous system disorder may be to blame. Severe, instant pain, and persistent or worsening headaches are worrying signs. A headache that becomes worse when you lie down may be a sign of raised pressure within the skull, and you should seek immediate medical attention.

- **Visual disturbance** Vision problems could simply be eyestrain, but they can also be telltale signs of an imminent problem. For instance, many migraine and epilepsy sufferers report seeing an aura around objects or bright flashes just before a migraine attack or a seizure. If you ever experience a loss of sight, even for only a few seconds, call your doctor immediately; such symptoms could be an early warning sign of stroke. Photophobia—when anything but dim light is painful—can be a sign of meningitis.

- **Memory loss** This can be hard to judge if it is only vague and generalized. Follow the criteria outlined under "Are your symptoms serious?" on page 51.

- **Altered sensation** Mild temporary numbness is not usually a cause for concern, but persistent numbness

---

IT'S NOT TRUE!

"Memory loss in old age means Alzheimer's"

With the increasing prevalence of Alzheimer's disease among older people, some people may misinterpret natural decline in memory function as a more insidious problem. Forgetfulness is a normal feature of advancing years, however. After the body turns 70, the connections between brain cells start to break up and slip to a mere 95 trillion—plenty to operate a healthy brain and nervous system, but function and reaction times do slow down.

can be a sign of nerve damage, for instance from multiple sclerosis or a complication of diabetes.

- **Physical weakness** If you suddenly experience weakness in any part of your body, you should see a doctor immediately. Paralysis of any sort, no matter how short lived, could be a sign of a transient ischemic attack (TIA), a minor stroke; this increases the likelihood of having a full-blown stroke within a year.

OTHER COMPLICATIONS

Certain long-term conditions put sufferers at a higher risk of neuro-logical problems. For example, people with diabetes mellitus or existing cardiovascular problems need to be particularly vigilant when it comes to neurological warning signs. Nerve damage—neuropathy—is a common consequence of poorly controlled diabetes: typical signs include numbness, weakness and pins and needles. Damage to the nerves that supply the eyes is also a risk in diabetics.

MENTAL SELF-AWARENESS

Being alert to signs of mental deterioration is often more difficult than looking out for a physical problem. Knowing the normal level of your abilities and the pattern of any fluctuations in these abilities may help you to spot anything out of the ordinary. Everyone is different in these respects, so it is hard to set general standards. To determine your own baseline of mental ability, try assessing your performance on mental exercises such as the ones on page 89. Also, think about other factors related to your neurological

well-being. Coordination and balance, for example, are heavily influenced by the health of your central nervous system.

Everyone experiences daily and even hourly fluctuations in levels of mental alertness and mood. Adults have a 90-minute cycle of alertness and drowsiness, for instance, which is superimposed on the 24-hour wake–sleep cycle. When you get tired or run down you can expect to forget things, become more clumsy, or simply slow down mentally. Bear this in mind when you think about or assess your mental capabilities.

Look at tomorrow's TV listings for one minute, and then close the paper and try to list as many of the programs, with their times, as possible.

Write a list of all the people with whom you are currently in contact, including their surnames where possible.

Write down the phone numbers of your ten closest friends or relatives.

A SNAPSHOT OF MEMORY SKILLS

Having a clear picture of your normal memory capabilities, both long and short term, can help you to set a benchmark for comparison later. Use the exercises in the bubbles to compare with the results you get in a few months or years time.

Make a list of what you had to eat for your last six meals.

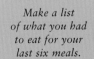

Adopt an anti-stroke lifestyle

Stroke is the number three killer in the developed world and a major cause of disability. The good news is that there are a number of highly effective steps you can take to guard against this potentially devastating condition.

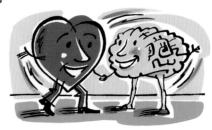

A health partnership—heart and brain
The health of your brain is closely linked to your heart's health. By looking after your heart, you reduce the risk of stroke.

When the blood supply to a part of your brain is interrupted or cut off, the tissue is starved of oxygen and can die—this is a stroke. A stroke can happen because a blood clot blocks one of the blood vessels supplying the brain or because one of these vessels bursts. In either case, the trouble is likely to have been caused by a problem with your cardiovascular health.

HEART HEALTH BASICS
Common cardiovascular problems include the clogging up of the arteries (atherosclerosis), high blood pressure, and diseased heart valves. In athero-sclerosis, the arteries become narrowed because of a build-up of fatty deposits made up of cholesterol and other material. Apart from making it easier for a blood clot to get stuck and block an artery—for example, the carotid artery—bits of these fatty deposits can break off and travel along the large arteries until they block a vessel that is too narrow for them to pass through.

High blood pressure increases the risk of narrowed arteries within the brain. Such vessels are not only

more likely to get blocked, but also more likely to burst, causing a hemorrhagic stroke. Heart valve problems carry similar risks—clots can form on the valve as the body responds to the damage, and clumps of these clots can break off, with devastating results.

PREVENTION IS KEY
You can play a large part in preventing a stroke by adopting an anti-stroke lifestyle. This may involve making changes in the way you live, but the rewards in terms of reduced stroke risk, improved general health, and increased energy will be well worth the effort. The first step is to identify your main risk factors.

The risk factors
The landmark Framingham Heart Study carried out by the National Hearth, Lung, and Blood Institute, identified the following cardio-vascular risk factors. Take note of factors that apply to you and focus on those you can impact.
- **Age** The older you are, the more you are at risk from both heart disease and stroke.
- **Gender** Men are more likely to develop heart problems, although women have a similar level of risk to men after menopause.
  - **Family history** If members of your family have had heart problems, your own risk of heart disease is increased.
  - **High blood pressure** Raised blood pressure—hypertension—is a particularly significant risk factor for stroke.
  - **Smoking** This is one of the leading risk factors for both heart disease and stroke.

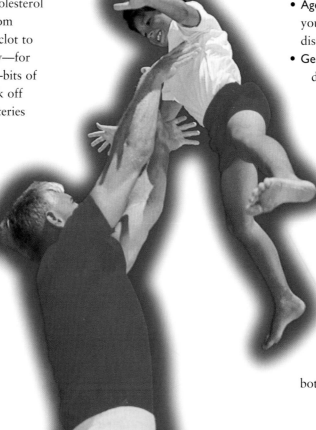

Zest for life
Keep fit and active: staying fit is one of the best ways to protect yourself from having a stroke in the future.

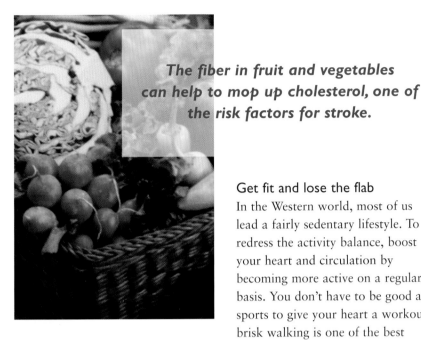

The fiber in fruit and vegetables can help to mop up cholesterol, one of the risk factors for stroke.

- **High blood cholesterol levels** High levels of total cholesterol and "bad" LDL cholesterol increase your risk.
- **Physical inactivity** Leading a lifestyle that makes few demands on your heart leaves it unfit and vulnerable to the risk of stroke.
- **Obesity** Being overweight puts extra stress on your heart and increases stroke risk.

MAKING CHANGES FOR LIFE

So now that you know the risk factors, what can you do to safeguard your heart and therefore your cerebral circulation? Some of the risk factors are out of your control (age, sex, family history), but there is still plenty of scope for taking action to improve the modifiable factors.

Give up smoking

Smoking impairs your cerebral circulation in a number of ways: it reduces the amount of oxygen your blood can carry, weakens the walls of your arteries, and raises your blood pressure. Not smoking is the single most effective measure you can take to protect yourself against stroke.

Get fit and lose the flab

In the Western world, most of us lead a fairly sedentary lifestyle. To redress the activity balance, boost your heart and circulation by becoming more active on a regular basis. You don't have to be good at sports to give your heart a workout: brisk walking is one of the best activities you can do. Current recommendations are to perform 30 minutes of moderately intensive activity at least five days a week.

Your brain will benefit within a few days from the raised oxygen levels and in the long term from the reduced risk of stroke.

Combining exercise with a low-fat diet is the best way to shed excess pounds and relieve the strain on your cardiovascular system.

Low-fat, low-salt equals low risk

Adopting an anti-stroke diet means eating foods that are good for your heart. To avoid raised cholesterol levels (or to lower high levels), keep your intake of saturated fats low. Consuming too much salt can contribute to high blood pressure, so watch your salt intake. Boosting your fiber intake, especially soluble fiber, slashes cholesterol levels, and this slow-releasing form of carbohydrate will ensure that your brain cells get energy all day long. As with any healthy diet, eating a range of fresh fruits and vegetables is essential for a balanced intake of cardioprotective antioxidants.

Alcohol in moderation

The old maxim "A little of what you fancy does you good" holds true for alcohol and heart health. Drinking a moderate amount of alcohol—wine, beer, or spirits are equally effective—on a regular basis can boost "good" HDL cholesterol and act on the body's clotting system to provide protection against heart attack and stroke. (See page 69 for sensible limits.) Excessive drinking and binge drinking, however, have a detrimental effect, raising blood pressure and causing palpitations and heart rhythm problems.

Which lifestyle factors are the most important?

Smoking is at the top of the list for anyone concerned about stroke: quitting cuts the risk of stroke in half. The effects of the other lifestyle recommendations are less, but still worthwhile. Taking up regular exercise relieves several risk factors. Exercise helps people who are overweight burn more calories, and boosts the body's metabolism, thus aiding with weight loss. Exercise also reduces blood pressure and cholesterol levels, as does drinking alcohol in moderation. Cutting down on salt intake is slightly controversial, but the general consensus is that we eat too much salt. Taken together, these additional factors could reduce your risk by a further 25 percent.

ASK THE EXPERT

Involve yourself in your healthcare

If you keep tabs on the health of your brain and nervous system, you are more likely to spot alarm signs early. An important part of being an active player in your healthcare is knowing when and for what to be tested.

You can be an active participant in the long-term care of your brain health, rather than a passive recipient of results and prescriptions. In order to do so, you need to know what check-ups and neuro-logical tests to expect from your healthcare provider.

CHECKS AND SCREENING

Neurological checks are done much less often than the more conventional tests for blood pressure or heart problems. But there are some standard tests of brain and nerve function that generally apply.

At birth, every newborn undergoes a thorough neurological examination to check that basic reflexes are present and in working order. Tests such as stroking the baby's cheek to produce a rooting reflex—turning the head towards the stroke—show that the nerve pathways between the spine and limbs are normal.

Developmental milestones

Normally, brain problems don't show up at birth. But as a child develops, it may become clear that his or her responses are not normal. In most cases, the more severe the problem, the earlier it becomes apparent. A child's developmental progress is assessed using a series of milestones—physical or mental achievements that occur in a predict-able order within a measurable time span. For instance, most babies have some control of head movement by the age of six weeks, but the head of a baby with cerebral palsy may still flop uncontrollably even at three months.

As the child grows up, the development of language comes to the fore: a precocious two-year-old might be speaking in fluent sentences, whereas an autistic child of the same age might have yet to utter a single word. Checks can pick up problems at an early age so that the least possible time is lost in normal development.

Learning difficulties

In the case of learning difficulties, attention disorders or dyslexia, the problem may not come to light until a child attends school. If your child

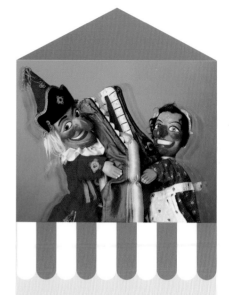

A bump on the head

You should get checked for concussion by a doctor after any episode involving a bang on the head that causes a loss of consciousness. While most knocks and bumps to the head are not serious, always see your doctor if you have double vision, if you vomit, or if you feel drowsy or confused after hitting your head.

is having trouble at school, is badly behaved and disruptive, or seems to have problems in some areas but not others (is very good at math, for example, but terrible at reading), it is worth discussing the situation with your child's teacher or doctor.

Your child may need to see a counselor or educational psych-ologist who can draw on a battery of different tests for diagnosing the specific nature of learning problems. Recognizing that your child has a problem is a positive step toward dealing with it. In many cases, properly tailored teaching techniques

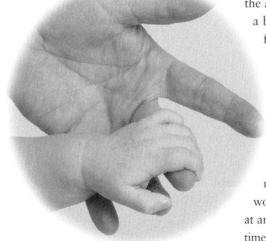

The reflex grip
A baby's ability to grasp a finger is one of the many reflex actions that are present from birth. These reflexes are a sign of a healthy nervous system.

can overcome or compensate for learning difficulties, helping children to be happier and better adjusted and possibly improving the quality of their education.

Screening for adults

While there are no specific neurological screening tests for adults, it is important that you have your cardiovascular health checked regularly; this impacts on your risk of having a stroke. Once you are over the age of 40, doctors advise that you begin having regular cardiovascular checkups. Generally speaking, healthy over-40s should have their blood pressure checked at least every five years. Cholesterol levels should be measured at the same intervals, but in women these tests are usually not necessary until after menopause.

Neurological tests are sometimes carried out if an elderly person is showing signs of confusion or if there is any question about his or her mental health. Doctors use various simple cognitive tests, which may include a series of questions designed to elicit orientation, memory and mental agility. For example, the person may be asked questions such as: "What day is it?" to check orientation, "Who is president of the United States?" to assess memory, and given a test of mental agility such as counting backwards from 100 subtracting 7 each time. Written tests, such as copying a drawing of a clock face, can also help a doctor to assess mental function.

HORMONES AND THE BRAIN

Right from the initial development of a baby's brain while still in the womb, hormones have a significant impact on the structure and function

Mobile phones: bad for the brain?

Mobile phones receive and transmit microwaves from the phone's aerial, and scientists believe that these microwaves, which are right next to the brain, can cause minute biological changes in the brain's electrical circuits. In adults at least, there is no evidence to suggest this will result in any particular problems. Children, however, may be more vulnerable because they have thinner skulls and their brains are still developing. Current advice is that children should avoid using mobile phones unless essential, until more research shows otherwise.

of the brain. The female sex hormone estrogen is believed to influence areas of the brain involved with thinking and memory, and researchers think the hormone acts on numerous sites within the brain. For instance, the hippocampus, a brain structure involved in memory

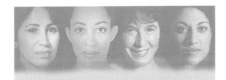

RESTORING MENTAL POWER WITH HRT

Hormone replacement therapy (HRT) helps to compensate for decreasing levels of estrogen and can relieve some of the mental symptoms of menopause, such as mood swings and loss of libido. HRT may also help to prevent memory from deteriorating. If your doctor thinks you may benefit from HRT, expect a period of experimentation while you find the best type of HRT, the optimum dose level, and best mode of delivery. HRT can be taken in the form of implants, topical applicators, capsules, and patches.

(see page 38), is rich in estrogen receptors, and the hormone has a significant effect on hippocampal levels of activity.

Menopausal impulses

During menopause many women have some problems in areas related to brain function as a result of the radical changes in hormone levels that occur at this time. Common consequences include mood changes, irritability, and depression. One survey has found that falling estrogen levels may be associated with a slight loss of performance in intelligence and memory tests. These changes in mental function are minor: even women whose estrogen levels fall early in life due to an early menopause still score better than men. But the findings do suggest another reason for women to be well informed about what is happening to them physically during the menopause and the possibility of hormone replacement therapy (HRT).

COMMON BRAIN HAZARDS

Potential threats to your brain can come from unexpected directions—even from the medicines you take to combat disease. How serious are such hazards, and what can you do to prevent them from affecting you?

Natural protection

Your central nervous system is cocooned, in biological terms, against the many dangers of the outside world. Several lines of defense shield the vulnerable nerve cells of your brain and spinal cord—the skull and spine, the meninges, and the cerebrospinal fluid.

Your natural defenses aren't protection against all possible hazards, however, and sometimes they need a helping hand from you. By being aware of the sources of potential risks to your nervous system, you can help to boost your brain health.

Medicines and your brain

Relatively few drugs cause brain-related side effects, thanks to the efficiency of the blood–brain barrier in keeping particular molecules from crossing over from the bloodstream into the central nervous system. But among those that do are some of the most widely used drugs in the world.

- **Oral contraceptives** Millions of women take oral contraceptives. These can trigger migraines, and some types (estrogen–progesterone combinations) very slightly increase the risk of stroke.
- **Painkillers** Analgesic, or pain-killing drugs, in the category of nonsteroidal antiinflammatories, such as ibuprofen and aspirin, can cause symptoms of confusion in the elderly. If you develop any side effects, your doctor should change the dose or prescribe an alternative. Keep your doctor informed about possible side effects and don't be afraid to raise concerns yourself.

Interfering with neurotransmitters

If your doctor diagnoses a neurological condition and prescribes medication, then be aware, as with taking any drug, that there are possible long-term adverse effects.

Certain drugs used to treat neurological disorders, such as those for psychiatric problems or Parkinson's disease, can themselves cause problems with mental function. For example, some antipsychotic drugs, such as haloperidol and fluphenazine, can cause symptoms that mimic those of Parkinson's disease—a phenomenon known as Parkinsonism.

In fact, most of the common drugs used to treat depression and schizophrenia carry a risk of central

Some drugs affect the brain within seconds. Inhaled drugs can pass into the bloodstream and cross into the brain tissue in as little as 15 seconds.

nervous system side effects, although these are usually minor. Tricyclic antidepressants and selective serotonin reuptake inhibitors can cause symptoms such as headache, tremor, and sedation.

Drugs for treating Parkinson's disease can cause psychiatric symptoms: for instance, long-term use of levodopa—a standard treatment for Parkinson's—can be associated with depression and psychosis. Such symptoms occur because the medication changes the delicate balance of neurotransmitters in the brain.

If you are caring for someone with Parkinson's disease or a psychiatric problem, be alert for the signs of side effects and work with the doctor to minimize or avoid side effects by changing drugs or altering doses.

Protect yourself against mental illness

Keeping yourself emotionally balanced is not always easy: As many as 23 percent of people in the U.S. suffer from a diagnosable mental illness in a given year. What can you do to keep your day-to-day life on an even keel?

Most people will, at some time in their lives, encounter depression, either in themselves, a partner, or a friend. It is, in fact, one of the most common illnesses in the developed world. And for many people the diagnosis of depression still carries a stigma.

DEPRESSED OR JUST LOW?

Mood can be viewed as a spectrum, with depression at one end and elation at the other. Everyone falls somewhere along this spectrum, and many people may find themselves at the depressed end at some time.

It is important to recognize that depression is a real illness that needs real treatment. If you know someone who has been feeling low for an extended period of time, or shows other symptoms such as constant fatigue, bouts of crying, feelings of hopelessness or despair, or morbid thoughts, don't assume that they simply need to pull up their socks. These feelings could be the physical manifestation of a chemical imbalance in the brain—drug therapy may be essential to redress this delicate

Some 70-year-olds perform better at tests of mental agility than some 20-year-olds; education and experience compensate for the deficiencies of aging.

balance. The ingredients in food can influence brain chemicals, so the problem could be something in a person's diet. Turn to page 83 to check out bad mood foods and refer to page 140 for more information about depression.

Anyone who feels low, and has done so for several weeks, should discuss their symptoms with their doctor.

CHANGING MEMORY

The ability to memorize, to learn new information, and to concentrate naturally declines as we get older, but this happens very slowly. For most of us, memories

remain a treasury that we will be able to dip into for the rest of our lives. Be proud of your treasury and pass on family stories to your children and grandchildren.

Seldom does the natural aging process cause serious problems with short-term memory until about the age of 70, beyond which some people experience a degree of difficulty with recalling recent events. This fall-off in immediate recall and mental flexibility is sometimes referred to by neurologists as "benign senescent forgetfulness"; it is not a dementia and for most people does not progress rapidly.

The best way to protect against mental deterioration is to exercise your brain on a regular basis. Turn to page 89 for some ways of giving your memory a workout.

THE TRIALS OF LIFE

Everyone experiences some symptoms of depression, anxiety, anger, or disappointment as short-lived responses to events in their lives. Some examples of these experiences are coping with losing or changing a job, the break-up of a relationship, or the death of a loved one.

The mood spectrum
We all experience variations in mood from time to time. Depression is one end of the spectrum, euphoria the other. In between there is a range of moods, usually a response to what's happening in our lives.

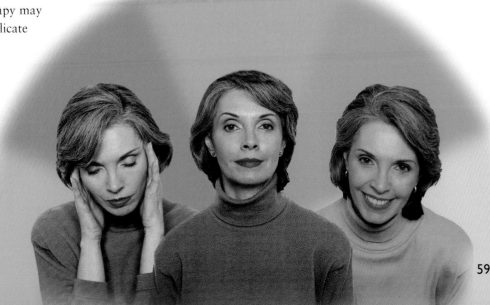

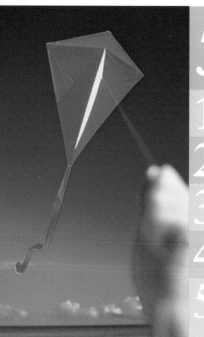

5 Ways to think positive

Changing from negative to positive ways of thinking can have a real impact on your emotional health.

1 Be kind to yourself. Don't listen to the critical negative voice in your head. Turn the negative volume down and crank up the voice that encourages you.

2 Keep things in perspective. Don't view situations in terms of absolutes, such as "awful" versus "excellent"—there is always a middle ground.

3 Don't label yourself or others. If you see yourself as "weak" and others as "strong" and "confident" you will always be the underdog. Human beings are fallible.

4 Don't always voice your fears. Try to think coolly when you are feeling pressured, and avoid using emotive language such as "I can't stand it" and "I can't do this."

5 Accentuate the good things. When someone asks you about your day, think about the things that have gone right and give them a higher prominence.

Too many traumas occurring in close succession can increase the likelihood of mental illness. The chance of succumbing to such stress is influenced in part by your genetic make-up, but your own thought processes also play a part. Even positive life events—such as being promoted or having a baby—can be stressful and precipitate depression.

Postnatal depression

About 85 percent of new mothers go through a spell of the "baby blues" three or four days after the birth. Feeling miserable, tearful, and irritable are typical symptoms, and we now know that new dads can have similar symptoms. Whatever the cause—changes in hormone levels, tiredness, or a feeling of anticlimax—it usually passes within days. Make sure that you get enough rest and ask your partner, family members, or friends to help take care of your new baby from time to time. Postnatal depression is a far more

serious condition. Mild depression turns to extreme anxiety about small things, along with feelings of inadequacy, tearfulness and a sense of desperation. If you think you may be suffering from postnatal depression, seek medical assistance as soon as you can because not only are you at risk of recurrent depression later in life, but your condition may also have a detrimental effect on your relationship with your child and on your child's development.

SEEING YOURSELF POSITIVELY

Psychologists have identified a number of "thinking errors" by which individuals magnify and reinforce the effects of stress by self-deprecation and critical thought processes. You can learn to stop negative thought patterns and reverse them with positive thinking techniques.

Learning how to see yourself and think about things in a positive way is like learning any skill—it requires

effort and practice. Eating healthily and exercising regularly will reduce your likelihood of developing physical illness and enhance your ability to cope with stress. Exercise has been shown to improve depression and reduce anger levels, so burn off your blues (see pages 86 to 87).

Most people feel happier about themselves if they are content with their own body image, but concern about how body weight should not become obsessive, as that could be a source of stress in itself.

Taking up or rediscovering a hobby or pastime can provide a distraction from your everyday problems; it is a useful way to unwind, broaden your horizons, and improve your self-esteem. Joining a club or group will get you out and about among like-minded people and will help to combat feelings of isolation.

KNOWING WHEN TO GET PROFESSIONAL HELP

Sometimes your own resources may not be enough, but help is available from many sources.

Your doctor is the first port of call and should provide a helpful, impartial ear. Discuss your feelings honestly; talk about how you feel about drug therapy and ask about counseling—your doctor will be able to refer you to a psychotherapist.

There are many different types of therapy available, including psycho-analytical therapy, behavioural therapy and counselling; each is valid in its own way, and your chances of successful treatment depend largely on whether you feel the therapy is right for you. It makes sense to explore the options and see which therapy suits you best.

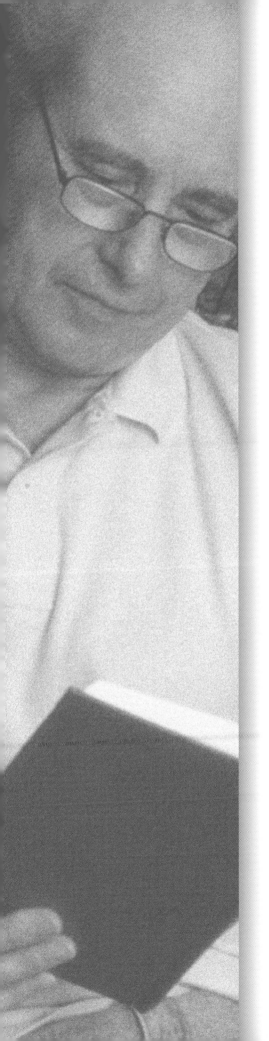

LIVE A BRAIN-HEALTHY LIFESTYLE

Depending on our lifestyle, we are all subject to situations that are potentially harmful to the brain. Experiencing stress, missing out on sleep, drinking too much alcohol, using recreational drugs, smoking cigarettes, loading up on caffeine—these can all have damaging effects on our brain health. Learning what happens to your brain in all of these situations puts you in the best position to take control and protect your brain from unnecessary harm. So, is yours a brain-healthy lifestyle?

63 *Learning to say "no" is an important part of keeping stress under control.*

66 *A good night's sleep is the key to a contented mind.*

69 *Even a couple of drinks over the recommended limit can damage your body's healthy equilibrium.*

72 *Not smoking is the biggest single step you can make to good brain health.*

74 *A few cups of tea or coffee can be mood enhancing, but overdoing the caffeine is a bad idea.*

Learning to handle stress

Whether you are tearing your hair out at work or caring for a sick relative at home, stress could be taking its toll on your brain and nervous system. Recognizing the signs and symptoms will help you to manage stress more effectively.

The word *stress* is derived from *stringere*, a Latin word that means "to press" or "to squeeze." It is now an everyday word—hardly a day seems to go by without hearing someone complain of being stressed out. What you may perceive to be a stressful situation, however, another person may not; how the mind responds to stress is completely individual. Our bodies, on the other hand, have predictable physiological reactions to stress—both in the short term and in the long term.

WHAT IS STRESS?

If you asked a selection of people to define stress, you could end up with as many definitions as the number of people quizzed. Researchers, however, describe it as the feelings and reactions you undergo when you perceive that the demands placed upon you exceed your ability to adapt physically or psychologically to those demands. So, whether or not you experience stress depends greatly on how well you think you are equipped to cope.

THE FIGHT-OR-FLIGHT RESPONSE

All of us must have experienced short-term stress at one time or another—be it an hour of suppressed panic during a meeting for which we are unprepared, or overstepping the curb on a busy street and having to jump back to avoid being hit by a car. A cascade of automatic body reactions goes into motion to safeguard you and prepare you for action—a throw-back to the so-called fight-or-flight response of our prehistoric ancestors:

- Blood is diverted to your brain (for quick thinking) and muscles (for a speedy getaway).
- Heart rate and breathing speed up to supply the brain and muscles with enough oxygen and glucose.
- Your pupils dilate to help improve your vision.

To produce almost instantaneous responses in your body, several biological systems work in cooperation: the brain and central nervous system, the hormone system, and the immune system.

During an acutely stressful situation, the hypothalamus deep within the brain activates the sympathetic nervous system. This in

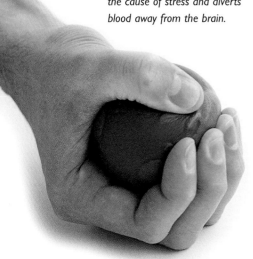

Squeeze to ease
The repeated action of squeezing a ball takes the mind away from the cause of stress and diverts blood away from the brain.

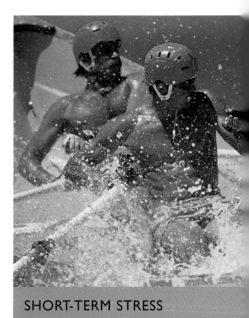

SHORT-TERM STRESS

Some people choose to exploit the thrill they get from the adrenaline rush of the fight-or-flight response; paradoxically, this is the same automatic reaction that is designed for their safety.

turn stimulates the adrenal gland to flood the body with chemicals called catecholamines—the best known is epinephrine—which are responsible for the fight-or-flight response. Sometimes, an awareness of these reactions can lead to a reinforcement of anxiety in a vicious circle.

UNDER LONG-TERM PRESSURE

If we are subjected to long periods of stress, such as becoming a full-time caregiver or having an extremely demanding and consuming job, the fight-or-flight response is taken over by a different physiological reaction.

When you are under prolonged stress, a complex series of hormonal changes occurs and transmitters in the brain undergo various alterations. Instead of involving the

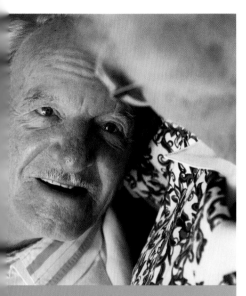

LONG-TERM STRESS

Often we don't think of taking on extra work or helping someone out as stressful, but the accumulative effect of such tasks combined with a lack of time for relaxation and rest soon shows.

sympathetic nervous system, the hypothalamus stimulates the nearby pituitary gland to prompt the release of different stress-related chemicals— called corticosteroids, such as cortisol—from the adrenal glands.

In the short run, cortisol mobilizes energy reserves, reduces inflamma- tion of body tissues, and enhances muscle tone so the heart can pump more nutrient-rich blood to the brain. Unlike the short-lived effects of adrenaline, however, the effects of cortisol are long lasting. In high concentrations, cortisol can directly alter the mood of an individual. Prolonged high levels have been shown to damage nerve cells in the hippocampus—part of the brain's limbic system involved in emotions, sexual behavior and memory— particularly if another hormone

called dihydroxyepiandrosterone is reduced. Receptors for cortisol are widely distributed through the brain, so the damaging effects of cortisol probably extend well beyond the limbic system.

When stress takes its toll

Emotionally taxing life events, such as bereavement or divorce, can lead to long-term psychological stress and in susceptible people can precipitate psychiatric illnesses such as depression or schizophrenia. Some researchers suggest that stress may also contribute to degenerative diseases of the brain such as Alzheimer's disease. How changes in the brain, in response to stress, may predispose someone to disease is still only incompletely understood, and further research is ongoing.

BECOMING YOUR OWN STRESS MANAGER

Whatever the cause of the tension you are experiencing, be it short term or long term, one of the best ways to relieve stress is to breathe deeply. According to research in both North America and Europe, breathing is linked to the release of neuropeptides—chemical messengers in the brain that make you feel good. The area of the brainstem involved in breathing contains a great many neuropeptides and neuropeptide receptors, so if you take a few moments to focus on your breathing and make your breaths deeper, your tension will give way to a sense of composure.

Making time

Now and again, most of us feel there just aren't enough hours in the day to get through everything that

Is there such a thing as good stress?

Experts link stress to all kinds of health conditions. But stress doesn't have to be bad for you. Some people actually enjoy a certain amount of stress and feel that it is good for them—it provides the incentive to meet deadlines and perform well. Positive stress from taking part in competitions or in new and exciting activities can also give you a real adrenaline high. Whether or not you perceive stress to be good or bad depends largely on the balance in your life: too little and your brain can become sluggish, leaving you feeling unmotivated; too much and you can easily become overstressed, exhausted, and unable to concentrate or focus on any task properly.

ASK THE EXPERT

we need to do. But often it isn't really a lack of time that is the problem, it's how effectively we use the time we have available.

Time management is a crucial aid to reduce stress in many situations and will give you more time for relaxation. If your stress is due to an overwhelming workload, you may need to change the way in which you approach your work. Try to tackle your tasks methodically, so that they don't "get on top of you"; make lists of your tasks, goals, and targets and prioritize them. Then you can see at a glance what you have to do and

FOR THE OVER-60s

Adjusting to a lack of stress

Negative mental images of particular situations or life events, such as associating retirement with the idea that your life as you know it is over, may become self-fulfilling prophecies. To counter any bad feelings, focus on replacing negative images with positive ones. Sort through all the pluses of retiring to see how positive an event it really is:

- **Pass Go!** Collect $200 and think of the time you have to devote to your passions, hobbies, and family.
- **Community chest** Congratulations! You have won a round-the-world cruise, and now you have the time to travel the globe experiencing life in other countries.
- **Chance** Now that your days are free, you can be spontaneous and forget about time restrictions.

- **Sports car** You can go for drives in the country whenever you want—you may even want to splurge on a new car.
- **A second home** It doesn't have to be Martha's Vineyard, but you may have enough free money now to buy a cottage in the country or a timeshare in the Caribbean.
- **Scottie dog** Consider getting a pet—not only is keeping a pet good for regulating blood pressure, but if you have a dog, the daily exercise will help to keep you physically and mentally active.

check off tasks as you complete them. Allow enough time for each task and do one thing at a time, completing each task before moving on. Say "no" to unrealistic demands. Misunderstandings can also make more work, so clarity when giving and receiving instructions is vital.

RIDING THE WAVES

The electrical activity of the human brain has a rhythmical quality that alters, depending upon its state of arousal. Alpha waves appear when your brain is alert but unfocused and your eyes are closed. Beta waves appear when your attention is focused and your eyes are open, such as when you are reading or working at a computer. These waves are faster, are produced more over the front portion of the brain, and are particularly prominent when you are active—especially when you are anxious or stressed. Your brain produces theta rhythms—slow rhythms—when you are drowsy and during light sleep. The theta state is often accompanied by unexpected dreamlike mental images.

The human brain is not designed to function at a constant level of

Fascinating rhythm
The frequencies of alpha, beta and theta waves illustrate the diversity of the brain's function at different conscious levels.

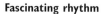 *alpha (relaxing)*

beta (concentrating)

theta (sleeping)

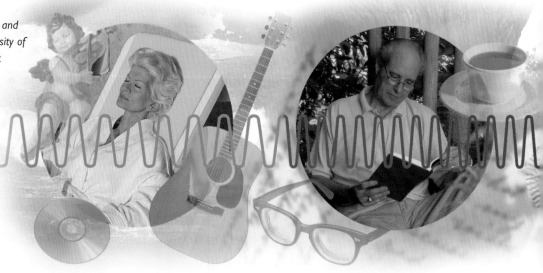

peak mental performance—it is much more efficient when periods of intense activity are broken by more contemplative and restful pursuits, such as listening to music. Music and rhythm can have profound effects on our emotions and moods, and some researchers have attempted to draw associations with the brain's underlying rhythmicity. Whatever the mechanism, listening to music has an undeniable link to the patterns of brainwaves. Upbeat music can uplift you and put you on a natural "high."

Studies have shown that listening to Mozart can make you more focused and productive, while tranquil "new age" sounds can help you to release tension and unwind.

So, try playing *Eine Kleine Nachtmusik* on your stereo on the commute to work to get your brain in gear, and see the difference; after a pressure-filled day, put on some ambient sounds and let your mind relax.

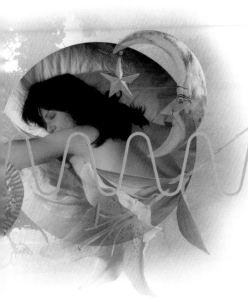

LEARN TO CALM YOUR MIND

From aromatherapy to yoga, relaxation techniques are numerous and most are very effective at reducing tension. Many people find that meditation works wonders for on-the-spot stress-relief, allowing them to empty their minds of the "business" associated with everyday activities and to reach a state of heightened awareness. Meditation need not be a religious or "spiritual" experience—though, for some people, it certainly is—you can simply use it as a practical tool to recharge your brain.

Transcendental tranquillity

Transcendental meditation (TM) involves slipping into a concentrated meditative state by repeating a phrase or mantra over and over in your mind. During this time, the brain produces alpha waves and any tension melts away. Research shows that people who regularly practice TM experience improved cognitive functioning and mental health.

Try this simple meditation exercise:
- Sit quietly in an upright position; you don't have to adopt the lotus position, a favorite chair is fine.
- Close your eyes and relax.
- Mentally repeat the word "peace" slowly and effortlessly—or choose your own mantra.
- Hear the word in your mind intermittently—don't concentrate too hard on the sound or meaning.
- Continue to repeat the word for 15 minutes. If your own thoughts or outside sounds distract you, take some deep breaths and gently bring your mind back to your mantra.
- Loosen your mind. You may find it difficult to focus at first, but with practice it will become easier.

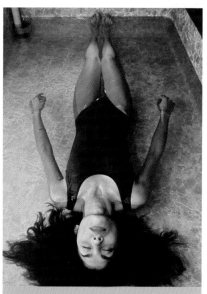

Flotation therapy

Why not immerse yourself in mineral-containing water and allow your body to become weightless in the minerals? A flotation tank or room is totally dark, there is no sound, you can feel nothing—sensory deprivation frees your mind.

The limbic system responds to flotation by inhibiting the release of hormones and neurotransmitters, such as epinephrine, norepinephrine, and cortisol, that in high levels can have a damaging effect on the brain. Floating also boosts the production of natural endorphins.

The brain produces slow, sleep-like theta waves during a flotation session. Often, floaters find that they have access to deep memories. Some people report suddenly remembering the strangest facts and experiencing wonderful clarity of thought.

Getting a good night's sleep

Sleep is an elementary process. We spend about a third of our lives asleep, and it seems to be essential for brain health, yet no one seems to know exactly why we need to sleep and how our bodies know when to sleep.

Sleep is the most conspicuous of the basic 24-hour cycles, or circadian rhythms, that govern our bodies. It is intricately tied up with the hormonal rhythms of growth, sexual maturation and reproduction, temperature regulation, and even feeding. The principal value of sleep may be to restore the balance between the neurological centers that are activated during wakefulness and to consolidate the processes of memory and learning—rather like rebooting a computer. Research also suggests that sleep has other roles, such as stimulating the immune

Time for bed
How much sleep we need changes throughout our lives, and general age-related patterns exist.

BABIES
A newborn infant may require as much as 20 hours of sleep per day, broken down into several sessions. This reduces to about 10 to 12 hours in early childhood—including an afternoon nap.

CHILDREN
The fact that babies and children need more sleep than adults backs up the idea that sleep is related to brain development. Sleeping time may be down to 9 or 10 hours a night by the age of 10.

THE ELDERLY
By late adulthood, 6 to 7 hours of sleep are usually sufficient, but with further aging sleep tends to become fragmented, and daytime wakefulness can be interrupted by spontaneous episodes of sleep or, naps.

ADULTS
In later childhood and adolescence, the adult sleep cycle of about 7 to 8 hours a day is finally established; although in some cultures an afternoon siesta is never abandoned.

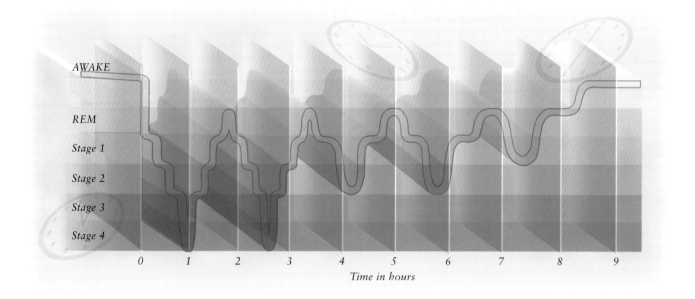

AWAKE

REM

Stage 1

Stage 2

Stage 3

Stage 4

0   1   2   3   4   5   6   7   8   9

Time in hours

system to protect against infections, cancers, and even aging. But why we need to "shut down" is still an unanswered question.

SLEEP STAGES

Sleep is not a passive event that occurs when the body is sufficiently tired but is an active biological process with several preprogrammed stages (see figure). Each stage of sleep has unique brainwave patterns and a number of physiological changes. The brain goes through a sequence of different waves during the night, including stages of rapid eye movement (REM) sleep—thought of as our "dream sleep."

THE MELATONIN FACTOR

The internal clocks that govern the daily rhythms of our bodies are controlled by a cooperative effort of various parts of the brain, including a group of neurons and projections at the base of the brain (the reticular activating formation) and the pineal gland. One of the functions of the pineal gland is to secrete melatonin— a potent sleep-inducing and sleep-maintaining hormone. Melatonin production is regulated partly by the

amount of light present (there are direct connections between the pineal gland and the retina of the eye) but also by the cycles of day and night. The winter blues—also known as seasonal affective disorder—may be caused by melatonin deficiency; some people find that exposure to bright light relieves their depression.

Work in harmony with your body rhythm by establishing a regular time to go to bed and to wake. During the day, an active lifestyle will ensure that you are physically fatigued, but strenuous activity close to the time you go to bed may be stimulating and prevent sleep. You should avoid caffeine-containing drinks close to bedtime (or longer if you're very susceptible to caffeine—see page 74), as caffeine delays sleep by reducing melatonin levels.

GETTING ENOUGH SLEEP?

U.S. researchers have recently sounded the alarm over rising levels of long-term overtiredness in the workforce. This is an increasingly common problem as escalating work demands and the attempt to juggle work, family, and social life put more and more pressure on finite time budgets.

Sleeping roller coaster

As well as dream or REM sleep, there are four stages of non-REM sleep: Stage 1 is the lightest; Stage 4 the deepest. You pass through each several times a night.

Melatonin for jet lag?

TALKING POINT

Traveling across time zones can lead to jet lag, a situation in which the body's time clock is "out of sync" with its surroundings. Some experts believe that jet lag is related to melatonin levels and that taking a supplement of melatonin helps to reset the body clock in the new time zone. So far, research has been inconclusive. Early tests found that melatonin did reduce jet lag, but a later trial using improved methods found that it made little difference.

If you do try melatonin supplements, avoid drinking alcohol, which has the same effect on the body as does melatonin, as the combination can produce unpleasant side effects.

Restricting sleep time leads to irritability, insomnia, depression, inability to concentrate, and generally poorer mental performance. With prolonged loss of sleep, reduced concentration and impaired coordination and judgment lead to more frequent errors. Eventually the brain's perception of the outside world can become so distorted that illusions or hallucinations occur. If you reach a state of extreme tiredness, the desire for sleep will probably become so intense that you'll fall asleep spontaneously during the day.

OVERTIREDNESS

Extreme tiredness is a leading cause of reduced productivity in the workplace. It is also a major cause of accidents on the road, in the home, and at work. Try to recognize when you are overtired and do not expect yourself to be able to cope without enough sleep—you will be much more efficient if you are rested and refreshed. See page 63 for some time-management tips, and set clearly defined timetables including adequate periods for rest and sleep. Try not to overburden your day with tasks that will eat into your leisure hours—it is vital to set aside some time to relax and unwind in preparation for sleep.

LIVING WITH INSOMNIA

Insomnia affects up to 40 percent of the population and is more frequently found in women and the elderly. With increasing age, the amount of sleep needed does reduce, but many people feel that they are not able to sleep as long as they need to, although only a fraction of those affected will ever visit their doctor for medical advice.

Identify possible causes

If you are finding it difficult to sleep, it could be because of a medicine you are taking. Some medications contain chemicals that disrupt the body's natural rhythms—ask your doctor if this could be the case and whether your prescription can be changed. Insomnia can also be a symptom of depression, which may need specific treatment and specialist advice, so don't suffer in silence—address the problem. As a short-term solution, your doctor may prescribe a sleeping medication. Bear in mind, though, that in the absence of psychological stresses and illness the human body will always get as much sleep as it needs.

EVERYDAY SLEEP STEALERS

The modern lifestyle can make it hard to get enough sleep. Juggling a career, a family, and household chores can leave little time to recharge batteries. Try to work out ways of increasing your sleep time.

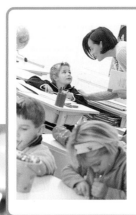

A mentally taxing day often provides no time for rest. Holding a position of responsibility can also mean having to work late in the office or having to do paperwork at home.

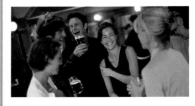

Evenings out with friends are important, but too many dinner dates and too much partying can take their toll on your brain health as they eat into your sleep time.

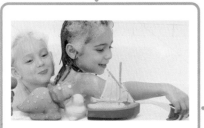

Young children are often early risers— so 6 A.M. starts are not unusual for parents with young families. Cleaning up after small children can be exhausting too.

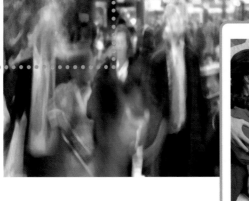

Keeping your relationship vital and healthy requires commitment, but setting aside quality time together often means that there is less time left over for sleep.

Alcohol and your brain

For most of us, social situations often involve an alcoholic drink or two, but how do our brains cope when alcohol's initial stimulating action rapidly transforms into a depressive one—Are we losing our minds?

As we take in that first glass of wine or bottle of beer, our brains reward us by increasing levels of the neurotransmitter dopamine. This gives us a stimulating and energizing buzz, but the pleasure doesn't last. The dopamine rush peaks after about 20 minutes and then—if we keep on drinking—it's downhill all the way.

Alcohol affects the nervous system in much the same way as an anesthetic: It depresses neurological activity by altering the properties of the brain cell membranes and the proteins attached to them, which are involved in the transport of calcium and in communication between cells. As more and more alcohol is consumed, the cerebral cortex, which rules part of the primitive brain (the limbic system), begins to lose its hold and the balance of power shifts.

SENSIBLE LIMITS
The recommended safe limits for alcohol consumption are 2 to 3 units a day for women and 3 to 4 units a day for men. One unit is 1 centiliter of alcohol, which is roughly equivalent to about 8 ounces of ordinary strength beer or one small glass of wine. About 30 percent of men and 10 percent of women exceed the recommended daily amount of alcohol on a regular basis.

There is no simple way to predict the level of alcohol in your bloodstream after drinking an alcoholic drink; it is affected by your sex, build, and liver metabolism. The effects of alcohol on the brain are influenced by the pattern of drinking as well as the quantity—long-term, high-level consumption is probably more harmful to the nervous system than episodic binge drinking, which in turn is more damaging than the one-glass-a-day approach.

A drunken brain consumes about 25 percent less glucose than a sober one, causing a dramatic reduction in neuronal activity.

LETTING YOUR HAIR DOWN
Most of us are familiar with the feelings of relaxation and confidence that accompany light drinking. But what happens as we continue to down a few more drinks? What is going on in the brain when speech becomes slurred, movement becomes clumsy, and balance is impaired?

After just one drink, one of the brain's major excitatory message pathways—the N-methyl-D-aspartate (NMDA)—becomes highly sensitized. This means that certain NMDA receptors are more easily activated by the neurotransmitter glutamate. The hippocampus, the cortex, and the nucleus accumbens (see page 30) are the most sensitized, heightening the thinking and pleasure-seeking parts of the brain—at least for a short period of time.

There comes a turning point, however, after which NMDA excitement wanes and the gamma-

---

IT'S NOT TRUE!

"Alcohol kills brain cells"

Are we losing valuable brain cells never to be recovered every time we drink alcohol? It is certainly no secret that alcohol can kill cells—it has been used as an effective disinfectant for hundreds of years. But you don't need to worry about killing brain cells if you drink sensibly: for that to happen you would have to drink 1000 times the legal limit for drivers. In regular excess, though, alcohol does become toxic.

aminobutyric acid (GABA)—a major inhibitory neurotransmitter in the brain—kicks in, stopping neurons from firing and dulling the activity in the brain. The cerebellum is highly affected, causing that telltale slur in the speech and uncertain feet.

Extremely high levels of alcohol slow down both the hippocampus, which adversely affects memory, and the thalamus, thereby throwing out a person's coordination and ability to control body movements.

OVERSTEPPING THE MARK

Alcoholism is a dependence on alcohol to such a degree that it interferes with health, relationships, and employment. The lifetime risk of becoming an alcoholic is 10 percent for men and 5 percent for women, but the mechanisms by which people become addicted are obscure and may involve a combination of genetic, psychological ,and cultural factors. Fewer than 20 percent of alcoholics are known to their doctors.

The grossly addictive nature of alcohol is best illustrated by the debilitating effects it has on the body when it is withdrawn. Tremors with associated nausea, sweatiness, flushing and racing heart can strike after only a short period of withdrawal from heavy alcohol consumption. In extreme cases, alcoholics may experience an alteration in their perception of events in their surroundings, such as hallucinations. Brainwave activity

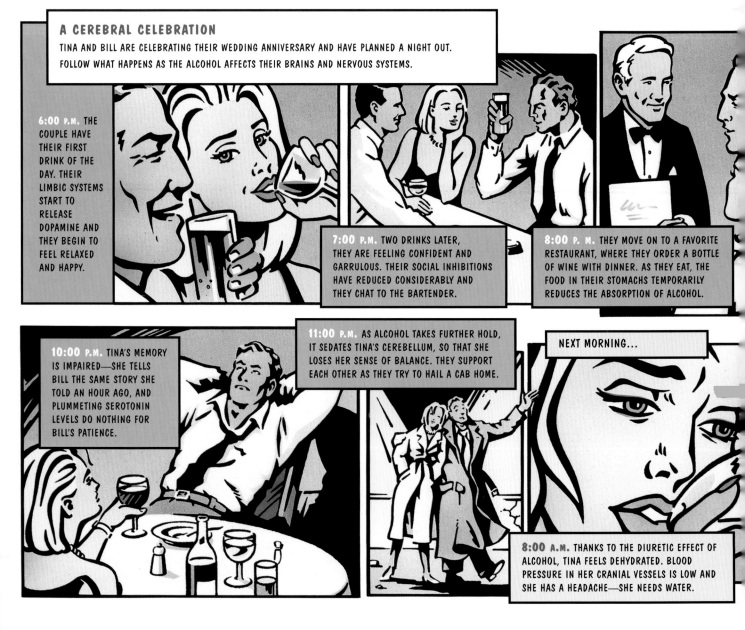

A CEREBRAL CELEBRATION
TINA AND BILL ARE CELEBRATING THEIR WEDDING ANNIVERSARY AND HAVE PLANNED A NIGHT OUT. FOLLOW WHAT HAPPENS AS THE ALCOHOL AFFECTS THEIR BRAINS AND NERVOUS SYSTEMS.

6:00 P.M. THE COUPLE HAVE THEIR FIRST DRINK OF THE DAY. THEIR LIMBIC SYSTEMS START TO RELEASE DOPAMINE AND THEY BEGIN TO FEEL RELAXED AND HAPPY.

7:00 P.M. TWO DRINKS LATER, THEY ARE FEELING CONFIDENT AND GARRULOUS. THEIR SOCIAL INHIBITIONS HAVE REDUCED CONSIDERABLY AND THEY CHAT TO THE BARTENDER.

8:00 P.M. THEY MOVE ON TO A FAVORITE RESTAURANT, WHERE THEY ORDER A BOTTLE OF WINE WITH DINNER. AS THEY EAT, THE FOOD IN THEIR STOMACHS TEMPORARILY REDUCES THE ABSORPTION OF ALCOHOL.

10:00 P.M. TINA'S MEMORY IS IMPAIRED—SHE TELLS BILL THE SAME STORY SHE TOLD AN HOUR AGO, AND PLUMMETING SEROTONIN LEVELS DO NOTHING FOR BILL'S PATIENCE.

11:00 P.M. AS ALCOHOL TAKES FURTHER HOLD, IT SEDATES TINA'S CEREBELLUM, SO THAT SHE LOSES HER SENSE OF BALANCE. THEY SUPPORT EACH OTHER AS THEY TRY TO HAIL A CAB HOME.

NEXT MORNING...

8:00 A.M. THANKS TO THE DIURETIC EFFECT OF ALCOHOL, TINA FEELS DEHYDRATED. BLOOD PRESSURE IN HER CRANIAL VESSELS IS LOW AND SHE HAS A HEADACHE—SHE NEEDS WATER.

may show abnormal rhythms and even epileptic discharges, which may lead to the development of a fit known by alcoholics as 'rum-fits'.

When a person consumes excessive amounts of alcohol on a regular basis, the alcohol acts like a toxin and leads to direct damage of muscle tissue, peripheral nerves and brain cells; damage to the latter is exacerbated by the poor diet of a typical alcoholic and, particularly, vitamin B deficiency.

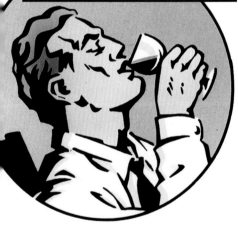

9:00 P.M. WITH MORE WINE, THE ALCOHOL'S DEPRESSIVE ACTION SPREADS, LABORING PROCESSES THAT REQUIRE COMPLEX NEURAL INTERACTION, SUCH AS SPEAKING AND WALKING.

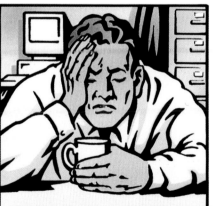

10.00 A.M. AFTER 10 HOURS' SLEEP, BILL FEELS GROGGY—ALCOHOL INTERFERES WITH THE NATURAL STAGES OF SLEEP. THE CAFFEINE IN A STRONG CUP OF COFFEE WILL PEP HIM UP A LITTLE.

What's the deal on drugs?

Illicit drugs have an enormous potential to affect the brain and nervous system both in the short and the long term.

Cannabis

For many people, cannabis has little effect and its actions may be dependent upon a person's mood, the situation in which it is taken and the strength of the sample. It is a depressant drug and a mild hallucinogen. An initial short-lived high is followed by a quieter phase of lethargy, poor memory, and impaired coordination.

Benzodiazepines

Medically prescribed drugs such as diazepam (Valium) or temazepam are used to relieve anxiety and to induce sleep. These drugs promote the activity of the neurotransmitter GABA, which inhibits electrical activity in the brain. This prevents the excessive brain activity caused by anxiety. Prolonged use can lead to dependence, and withdrawal can result in severe attacks of anxiety.

Amphetamines and Ecstasy

By promoting the production of the excitatory chemical norepinephrine, amphetamines cause overarousal and hyperactivity. As the effects wear off, users become irritable, tired, and anxious, and prolonged use can lead to paranoia and hallucinations. Ecstasy—a related drug—produces feelings of euphoria and extreme overactivity, which can lead to raised body temperature, dehydration, and, very rarely, sudden death.

Cocaine

A stimulant drug, cocaine is similar to the amphetamines in its actions on the nervous system, producing overarousal and euphoria— potentially making it an extremely addictive drug. Its withdrawal can lead to severe physical discomfort, with symptoms of panic, depression, lethargy, and an intense craving for the drug.

LSD

One of a group of drugs that became known in the 1960s as the "psychedelics," LSD distorts the brain's perception of the world. It is a synthetic drug, but similar agents do occur naturally as poisons in certain plants—for example in "magic" mushrooms and the peyote cactus. All "psychedelics" can produce mood swings and delusions and may provoke lasting psychotic disturbance.

Opioids—morphine and heroin

These agents were first derived from the juice of the opium poppy. The main components are morphine and diamorphine (heroin)—narcotics that block the transmission of pain signals within the brain. In medicine, opioids are invaluable as painkillers and as anxiety-reducing drugs in painful or terminal illnesses. Recreational users choose to take opioids as they produce intense feelings of pleasure. Opioids are highly addictive and have withdrawal symptoms that include cramps, vomiting, diarrhea, and intense cravings. On occasion, taking illegal opioids can be fatal.

Resisting nicotine addiction

Smoking has complex and addictive effects on the brain's chemical signaling mechanisms. By interfering with neurotransmitters, nicotine gets smokers "hooked" and makes it very difficult for them to give up the habit.

In the Western world, almost one in five deaths is smoking-related. But despite such shocking statistics, many people—by age 19, about 20 percent of the U.S. population—continue to smoke, because they are addicted to nicotine. Research suggests that some people are genetically predisposed to nicotine addiction through subtle differences in their brain chemistry.

THE NICOTINE RUSH

At first glance, cigarette smoking seems to have a beneficial effect on the brain. Nicotine has a mood-elevating effect by interfering with levels of the chemical dopamine in the brain. It inhibits the production of the enzyme monoamine oxidase, which breaks down dopamine and the neurotransmitter norepinephrine. So by reducing the levels of enzyme, nicotine effectively increases the levels of dopamine, leading to better psychological performance and enhanced attention. But when the effects of nicotine wear off, monoamine oxidase levels return to normal, which reduces the levels of the feel-good dopamine— starting a vicious

circle where nicotine is used to lift mood and relieve depression.

High nicotine levels also lead to increases in the number of receptors for acetylcholine—an important signal-transmitting chemical between brain cells with a role in memory and attention. As seen below, however, it is a side effect of this action that reinforces the smoking habit and contributes to addiction.

SMOKE AND STROKE

The attractions of smoking pale into insignificance in the face of the dangers associated with the habit. Smoking is a major risk factor for stroke. The mechanisms by which smoking causes strokes are many and include an increase in heart disease and the clogging up of large arteries such as the carotid artery, which

takes blood to the head and neck. Levels of cholesterol in the bloodstream are higher in smokers and the clotting cells or platelets are more "sticky." Smoking may directly damage a vessel's lining, making it more likely to become blocked, and the high levels of carbon monoxide in the blood may also lessen the ability of brain cells to use oxygen. Brain scans of smokers can reveal severe damage to neural pathways deep inside the brain as a result of smoking.

Chain smoking
The mimicking action of nicotine leads the smoker from one cigarette to the next: a vicious circle.

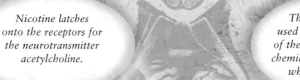

The nicotine stimulates the receptors far more than acetylcholine, wearing down their sensitivity.

Nicotine latches onto the receptors for the neurotransmitter acetylcholine.

The receptors get used to the high levels of the acetylcholine-like chemical and crave more when levels drop.

TELL YOURSELF YOU WANT TO QUIT

Withdrawal symptoms from nicotine include a craving for cigarettes, plus irritability, anxiety, increased appetite, and weight gain—not an attractive prospect. But help is at hand.

Nicotine replacement

The main focus of smoking for your brain is the effect of nicotine—if you can wean yourself off this drug, then you've kicked the habit. To beat the cravings, you can reduce your fix using nicotine replacement—a skin patch, inhaler, chewing gum, or even a nasal spray. Everyone is different, so try a few devices until you find what works best for you. You may continue to experience some cravings for a while, but they should be of a more tolerable level.

It's a strike!

By filling your free time with non-smoking–related activities, you can reprogram your mind to relax in a healthier way.

Motivational mind power

Remember, though, that using nicotine replacement is most likely to be successful if you are really committed to quitting—just sticking on a patch and crossing your fingers won't work. Success depends on a combination of willpower, support from friends and family, and a little behavioral therapy (see right).

SECOND-HAND SMOKERS

Passive smokers are exposed to the same noxious substances in exhaled cigarette smoke as regular smokers and have an increased incidence of stroke and cancer when compared with the nonsmoking population. Carbon monoxide levels in the blood can be elevated to similar levels to regular smokers, so the brain could be receiving less oxygen. Because there is very little nicotine in exhaled smoke, however, passive smoking is not addictive—so passive smokers have all the pain associated with smoking and none of the pleasure.

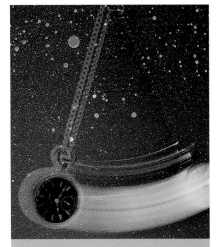

Retrain your mind

There is no such thing as a quick-fix, no-nonsense quit-smoking technique that works for everyone. Here we focus on how your brain can help you to reach the smoke-free zone.

- **Change your behavior** If you associate having a cigarette with working late to meet a deadline, for instance, you have to change that link in your mind. Instead of rushing out for a cigarette break, walk around the block and breathe deeply to clear your head.

- **Visit a hypnotherapist** In a session, your conscious mind is distracted while the hypnotherapist talks to your subconscious mind, suggesting how wonderful a nicotine-free life will be. Positivity and resolve are instilled in you and these feelings remain once the session is over. Although anyone can be hypnotized, it is not successful for everyone—you need to want to quit.

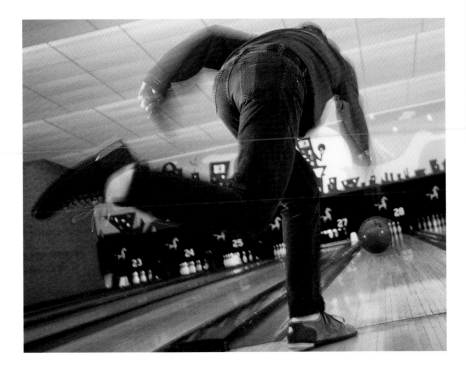

Caffeine—not just a coffee issue

Caffeine is the most widely consumed drug in the world and its consumption occupies a central place in many cultures. Some doctors feel, however, that its potential to produce harmful effects should make us more wary.

Caffeine not only inhibits phospho-diesterase (an enzyme that regulates cellular energy) but it also blocks the receptors for adenosine, a chemical that decreases excessive brain activity. Caffeine's interference allows the brain's stimulants—glutamate and dopamine—to rule the show.

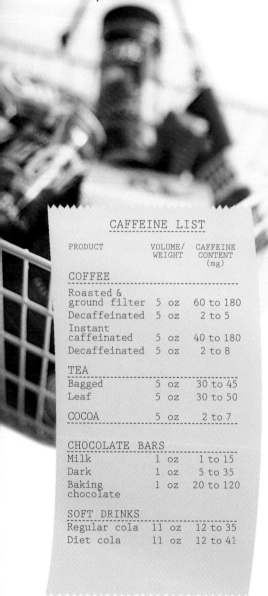

CAFFEINE LIST

PRODUCT	VOLUME/ WEIGHT	CAFFEINE CONTENT (mg)
COFFEE		
Roasted & ground filter	5 oz	60 to 180
Decaffeinated	5 oz	2 to 5
Instant caffeinated	5 oz	40 to 180
Decaffeinated	5 oz	2 to 8
TEA		
Bagged	5 oz	30 to 45
Leaf	5 oz	30 to 50
COCOA	5 oz	2 to 7
CHOCOLATE BARS		
Milk	1 oz	1 to 15
Dark	1 oz	5 to 35
Baking chocolate	1 oz	20 to 120
SOFT DRINKS		
Regular cola	11 oz	12 to 35
Diet cola	11 oz	12 to 41

STIMULATING YOUR MIND
The effects of caffeine can vary enormously from one person to another, partly because of genetic differences in the speed with which it is metabolized. On average, the stimulating effects of a cup of coffee take five to six hours to wear off, though for women taking oral contraceptives the effects last twice as long and for smokers half as long.

Caffeine also acts more specifically on the limbic system, which regulates emotion, mood, and circadian rhythms, such as the sleep–wake cycle. Just one cup of regular coffee in the morning contains enough caffeine to energize you, make you more active, put you in a good mood, and improve your concentration. The same cup at night would keep you awake and reduce the quality of sleep when you do drop off.

A SLAVE TO CAFFEINE?
We all need a pick-me-up now and again and caffeine-containing drinks, foods, and pills usually give us the lift we need to keep us ticking over. Relying on caffeine, though, can be damaging and it is well worth keeping tabs on your intake. The physical effects of missing caffeine can include irritability, anxiety, fatigue, tremor, nausea, and

Check out the caffeine levels
Cast your eye over the caffeine "shopping list"; you may be surprised to find out how much caffeine you unknowingly consume.

moodiness, but headache is the most common complaint. In some people, symptoms can occur only a couple of hours after missing a usual morning coffee. You may have experienced the Saturday morning headache that follows high caffeine intake at work and then relative abstention at home.

CAFFEINE LIMITS
An average worldwide caffeine consumption is about 75 mg per person per day, but this soars as high as 200 mg in the U.S. and the U.K. and up to 400 mg in Sweden and Finland. Caffeine metabolism varies among individuals and so it is difficult to establish a "dose" at which people experience adverse effects; ongoing research aims to identify a healthy limit. Doses exceeding 30 mg per kg body weight, though, are likely to be harmful—equivalent to about 9 cups of strong coffee for a 126-lb woman and about 11 cups for a 154-lb man.

Are there any drawbacks to taking caffeine pills or drinks to stay awake?

An occasional caffeine pill or drink works wonders when you need to stay awake, perhaps during a night-time drive. Arousal levels can become excessive with excess use, though, interfering with concentration and performance. Even brief exposure to high doses may lead to withdrawal symptoms, which tempt you to increase your dosage.

ASK THE EXPERT

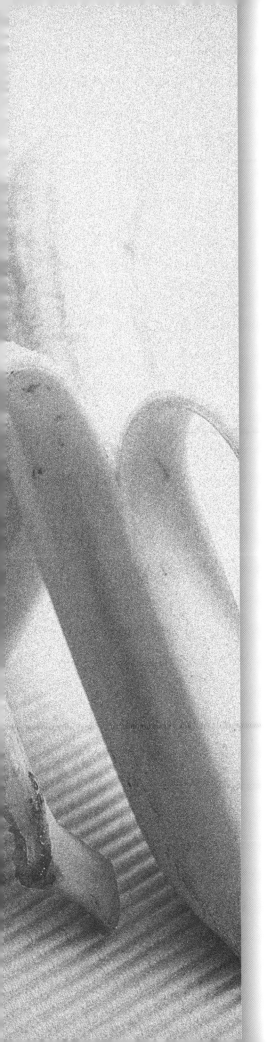

EAT A BRAIN-HEALTHY DIET

You are what you eat, and as far as your brain is concerned this is certainly the case. Your food choices—what, when, and how much you eat—can have far-reaching implications for your brain function and your mood. Your brain needs a variety of nutrients, vitamins, and minerals in order to function efficiently, and by making sure you strike a healthy dietary balance, you can benefit from its optimum function. Learn, too, how to use foods positively: to revitalise your energy levels, to beat stress, and to enhance your well-being.

76 *There's a lot of truth in the old saying "fish is brain food." Find out how a tuna sandwich can work wonders to enhance your brain function.*

80 *Did you know that eating little and often keeps the brain operating at its peak?*

82 *Learn how foods influence your brain's chemistry—a bad mood could be caused by something you ate.*

Food for thought

Foods have a huge range of health-giving properties for all parts of the human body, the brain being no exception. With a little nutritional know-how, you can boost your mental activity and make the most of your genetic potential.

Most of us are aware of the importance of eating a balanced diet, but what does this really mean in terms of brain health and function—what should we be feeding our minds?

PROTEIN, THE BASIC BUILDING BLOCK

The brain's signaling chemicals—neurotransmitters—are dependent on a good supply of protein. Protein is also necessary for the growth and maintenance of every cell in the human body, and it provides 10 to 15 percent of our total dietary energy requirements. Generally speaking, we normally eat more protein than we need: The average healthy man needs approximately 2 ounces of protein each day and the average healthy woman 1½ ounces each day. An 8 ounce portion of steamed salmon would provide this daily requirement, but for your body and brain to work well, you need to eat protein from different sources every day. This isn't hard to do, since protein is found in many foods—meat, fish, eggs, milk, cheese, yogurt, potatoes, nuts, legumes (peas, beans, lentils), and cereals (rice, wheat, oats and bread).

Essential amino acids

Proteins are made up of amino acids—compounds containing carbon, hydrogen, oxygen, and nitrogen—the elements necessary for life. There are more than 20 amino acids that, combined in different sequences, make up the many types of protein

your body requires. Eight amino acids are known as essential amino acids because your body cannot manufacture them, so they have to be supplied through your diet. If your diet contains foods with the right mixture of essential amino acids (from a variety of proteins), then your body can use them as building blocks to synthesize all the others.

Amino acid disorders

Certain metabolic disorders can affect the brain and nervous system. Phenylketonuria is an inherited disorder in which the enzyme responsible for converting the amino acid phenylalanine into another

amino acid, tyrosine, is defective. If it goes undetected, phenylalanine builds up in the body, resulting in mental retardation and brain damage. Fortunately, this condition is rare and screening tests have been designed to detect it at birth.

Some researchers have linked amino acids with epilepsy. Sixty percent of epilepsy sufferers have a reduced ability to synthesize the neurotransmitter gamma-amino-butyric acid (GABA), for which amino acids are essential. Research to examine the effects of dietary changes on epilepsy is ongoing and may reveal whether diet can influence this condition.

CARBOHYDRATES TO FUEL YOUR BRAIN

During digestion, carbohydrates are converted into glucose, which is stored in the body in a form called glycogen. Glucose and glycogen act as fuel for all the body's processes, including brain activity. Unlike muscles, the brain can store only very small amounts of glycogen, so it is vital that you ensure a regular supply of glucose to keep your brain working at its peak.

Slow-release starches

Starchy foods—complex carbohydrates—should form the basis of each meal and snack. Many people still believe that starchy foods such as bread, potatoes, rice, and pasta are fattening and should therefore be avoided. In reality, these foods are sources of complex carbohydrates, nutrients that should supply just over half of our daily energy intake.

Complex carbohydrates are broken down by the body slowly to provide a steady supply of glucose, unlike

---

How do vegetarians maximize intake of brain food?

If you don't eat animal products, it is still possible to obtain all the essential amino acids from the right combinations of plant sources, such as nuts, soybeans, legumes (peas, beans, and lentils), cereals, and seeds. However, as vitamin B_{12} is found almost exclusively in animal products, you should eat fortified cereals, yeast extract and seaweeds for vitamin B_{12}, because it is vital for the myelination of nerve cells—a deficiency can lead to numbness and tingling.

ASK THE EXPERT

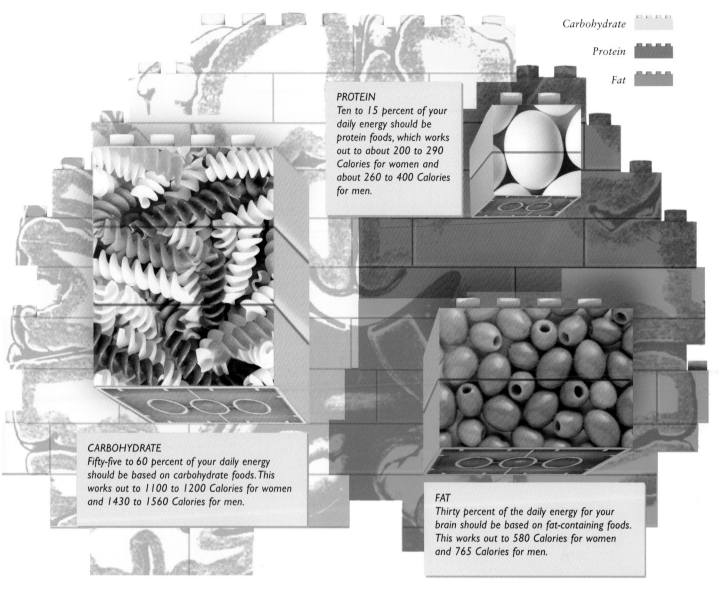

Carbohydrate

Protein

Fat

PROTEIN
Ten to 15 percent of your daily energy should be protein foods, which works out to about 200 to 290 Calories for women and about 260 to 400 Calories for men.

CARBOHYDRATE
Fifty-five to 60 percent of your daily energy should be based on carbohydrate foods. This works out to 1100 to 1200 Calories for women and 1430 to 1560 Calories for men.

FAT
Thirty percent of the daily energy for your brain should be based on fat-containing foods. This works out to 580 Calories for women and 765 Calories for men.

Building brain power
Eat from the three food groups to meet your daily energy requirements to ensure your brain is working at optimal capacity.

simple carbohydrates (sugars), which are absorbed quickly and can lead to rapid highs and lows in blood glucose levels. Sources of complex carbohydrates include bread, breakfast cereals, tortillas, chapatis, pasta, rice, potatoes, yams, starchy root vegetables, fruit, and legumes.

Choosing a breakfast of toast or cereal in the morning will ensure a good carbohydrate start to your

day, and this can be followed by potato salad, chili bean burritos, or brown rice for later meals. On the whole, unrefined "brown" versions of starchy foods are better for adults than the white ones because they retain most of their original nutrients. It is different for children, however, because if they fill up on too much fiber they may not be getting enough of the energy-dense foods they need.

Eastern promise
A typical Indian diet, based on rice, potatoes, yams, chapatis and poppadoms, comprises all the slow-release carbohydrates the brain requires for healthy function.

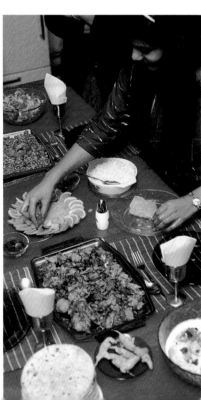

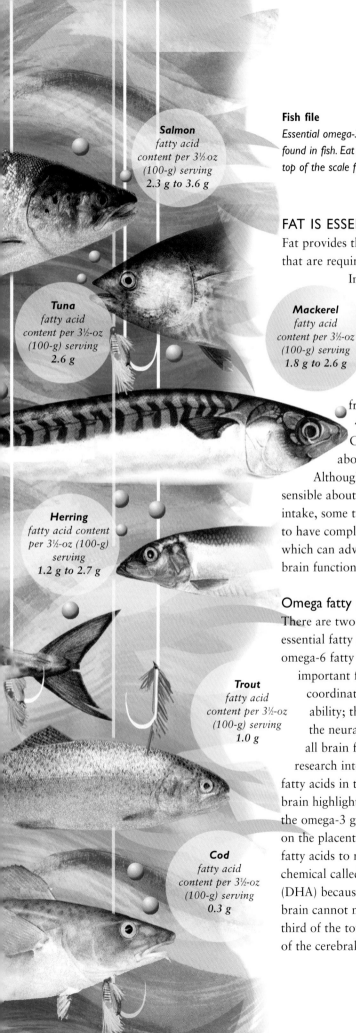

Salmon
*fatty acid
content per 3½-oz
(100-g) serving
2.3 g to 3.6 g*

Tuna
*fatty acid
content per 3½-oz
(100-g) serving
2.6 g*

Mackerel
*fatty acid
content per 3½-oz
(100-g) serving
1.8 g to 2.6 g*

Herring
*fatty acid content
per 3½-oz (100-g)
serving
1.2 g to 2.7 g*

Trout
*fatty acid
content per 3½-oz
(100-g) serving
1.0 g*

Cod
*fatty acid
content per 3½-oz
(100-g) serving
0.3 g*

Fish file

Essential omega-3 fatty acids are mainly found in fish. Eat plenty of those fish at the top of the scale for optimum brain health.

FAT IS ESSENTIAL

Fat provides the essential fatty acids that are required for brain function. In recent years there has been a lot of publicity encouraging people to eat less fat. In real terms, this means reducing fat intake from today's average of 40 percent of total Calories from fat to about 30 percent.

Although a lot of people are sensible about reducing their fat intake, some take it too far and try to have completely fat-free diets, which can adversely affect healthy brain function.

Omega fatty acids

There are two main groups of essential fatty acids: omega-3 and omega-6 fatty acids. The former are important for healthy vision, coordination, and learning ability; the latter form part of the neural tissues and influence all brain function. Ongoing research into the role of essential fatty acids in the development of the brain highlights the importance of the omega-3 group. A fetus depends on the placental uptake of omega-3 fatty acids to make an essential chemical called docosahexanoic acid (DHA) because the fetal liver and brain cannot make enough. Up to a third of the total fatty acid content of the cerebral gray matter in a fetus is DHA. The retina in the eye also has a high concentration of this chemical, so make oily fish a regular weekly feature in your diet.

Sources of omega fatty acids

Omega-3 fatty acids are derived from linolenic acid, found in rapeseed oil, soy bean oil, spinach, and oily fish such as herring, mackerel, trout, sardines, and salmon. Omega-6 fatty acids are derived from linoleic acid (not to be confused with linolenic acid), which can be found in vegetable oils, such as sunflower oil and olive oil. Adults need about 1 to 2 grams of the omega-3 fatty acids per day (approximately 2 teaspoons of rapeseed oil or a 3½ ounce portion of herring) and ⅛ ounce of the omega-6 fatty acids (2 teaspoons of sunflower oil) each day. To make sure you are getting enough of these healthy oils, snack on some soybeans or whole grain bread, or else make your own dressing with rapeseed or olive oil and add to a leafy green salad accompanying your main meals.

Animal fats

As for meat, cheese, cream, and butter, the fat in these is high in cholesterol and can contribute to cardiovascular disease. To give your brain a boost, try cutting down on these foods and substituting vegetable oils and oily fish.

MIRACLE MICRONUTRIENTS

The brain needs more than just protein, carbohydrates, and fat; a good supply of micronutrients—vitamins and minerals—is also essential for healthy nervous system function. A balanced intake of all the vitamins is vital, but with the exception of B$_{12}$ (see below) and folate (folic acid, see page 80), no one vitamin stands out in relation to brain function; here instead we will concentrate on minerals.

Sodium

More commonly eaten as sodium chloride or salt, sodium regulates nerve and muscle function and, together with potassium, maintains the fluid balance in the body's cells and tissues. In the Western world, most people eat too much salt, so it is unusual for people to experience a sodium deficiency.

Potassium

Working in harmony with sodium, potassium is essential for the transmission of nerve impulses, and early signs of deficiency are usually apathy and weakness. Most plant

Go bananas!
Packed with potassium, bananas are great snacks for keeping your nervous system operating at peak performance.

foods are good sources of potassium: bananas, nuts, seeds, legumes, avocados, wholegrains, dried fruit, tomatoes, and potatoes, so think of these when you're lacking in energy and you need a snack.

Calcium

Good calcium intake is essential to promote efficient functioning of nerves and muscles; it is involved in the conduction of electrical impulses along nerve cell axons. A deficiency—also called hypocalcemia—can manifest itself in muscle twitching and general fatigue. Great sources of calcium include milk and milk

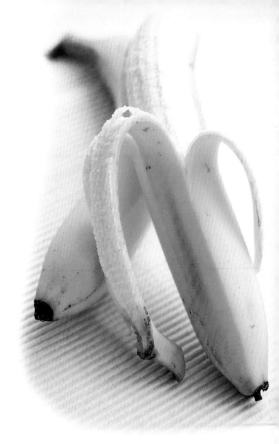

products, dark-green leafy vegetables, canned sardines, and salmon.

Magnesium

This mineral is important for the proper function of the hippocampus, a part of the limbic system that regulates mood and controls memory and learning. Good sources are nuts, dried apricots, dried figs, oatmeal, wholemeal flour, and yeast extract.

Iron

This mineral is essential for the formation of hemoglobin in red blood cells, a vital substance that carries a constant supply of oxygen to the nutrient-greedy brain. An adequate iron intake can improve mental function and academic achievement. Watch out for early signs of iron deficiency—fatigue and lack of concentration. Meat, sardines, egg yolks, and dark-green leafy vegetables, such as spinach, are all excellent sources of iron.

° **FOR THE OVER-45s**

B$_{12}$ for lifelong brain function

Nutritional experts have suggested that a healthy intake of vitamin B$_{12}$ might prevent or reverse the decline in cognitive functioning associated with the aging process.

As you age, your stomach produces less acid to break down and digest food to release its nutrients. The uptake of vitamin B$_{12}$ depends on a protein called "intrinsic factor," which is produced by the acid-making cells.

Dementia, in particular, can be caused by a B$_{12}$ deficiency and studies suggest the condition may improve by taking a monthly supplement of vitamin B$_{12}$.

Vitamin B$_{12}$ and folate—another B vitamin—are both essential in the synthesis of DNA, which is a central component of all cells.

Older people who no longer have to cook for a family or who live on their own can sometimes get bored preparing meals and may subsist on a nutritionally poor diet. People with inadequate diets like this are likely to have a folate (folic acid) deficiency, which can lead to depression and even dementia. A diet containing plenty of green leafy vegetables, nuts, grains and liver will ensure a healthy supply of folate.

Feeding the brain

Your brain is an energy-hungry organ—it may make up only 2 percent of your total body weight, but it uses up to 30 percent of your daily calorie intake. Providing your brain with a healthy diet will improve its function.

Your own information superhighway contains 100 billion nerve cells; each of these needs a continual supply of food (as glucose) and oxygen. Oxygen is in the air we breathe, but we have to eat to get glucose to keep our brains functioning properly. Everything you do, even something sedentary such as reading this book, involves activity in your brain, which uses up vital energy. Your brain never stops—even while you sleep your brain is still active, processing information and controlling body functions.

Even at rest, your brain grabs 20 percent of your body's blood glucose— and you wonder why you're feeling grouchy first thing in the morning:

Your brain is hungry and if you don't feed it, you'll drain its power. Studies done at the National Institute of Mental Health in Bethesda, Maryland, have shown that a healthy diet does benefit your brain and its functioning, and below we take it one step further and look at how to use food through the day to take advantage of your brain's natural "state of mind."

FOOD AND THE BRAIN THROUGH LIFE

It's never too late to start eating a "healthy brain" diet, but ideally this should begin before conception. As a woman, your chances of conceiving are much better if you and your partner are both eating a wide variety of foods, and if you are at the higher end of the healthy weight range. The USDA now recommends that women of childbearing age consume 400 mcg supplement of folic acid daily, to help to prevent neural tube defects, such as spina bifida. This amount can be in supplement form or eaten as part of a balanced diet that includes green leafy vegetables, legumes, citrus fruits and juices, and most berries. Between conception and birth, the rate of new nerve cell production in a growing baby averages 250,000 neurons a minute. There is rapid synthesis of brain tissue during the last trimester of pregnancy and in the first few weeks after birth. Part of this development involves complex lipids (fats) being formed from essential fatty acids, which are found in breast and formula. It is good to know that our first food in life gives our brains the best possible start.

BOOST YOUR BRAIN THROUGHOUT THE DAY

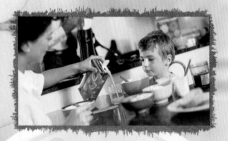

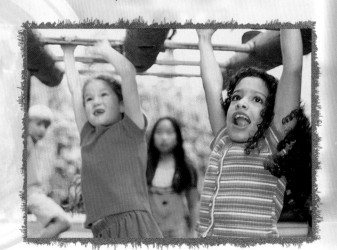

MID-MORNING *According to research, people who have eaten a cooked breakfast can feel more contented, interested, sociable, and outgoing than those who have had cereal and toast for breakfast or had no breakfast at all.*

BREAKFAST *After the night's mini-fast, cereal with milk and a banana or a cooked breakfast such as smoked salmon and scrambled egg are both brain-healthy options. Skipping breakfast affects memory, as the brain misses its glucose boost.*

LUNCH *Too much carbohydrate can cause tiredness, so a protein-based lunch will help to boost attention span for an afternoon's work. Avoid large meals in the middle of the day; they divert your blood supply from your brain to your digestive system, making you drowsy.*

At birth, your brain weighs less than 1 lb (450 g) and contains all the nerve cells you will ever have; by the time you are a fully grown adult, your brain has tripled in weight and quadrupled in size.

Energy for growth and learning

Development of the nervous system and brain is largely in place by about two years, and from this time into childhood and adolescence, the most important aspects of diet for a healthy brain are energy and fatty acids. A balanced diet rich in energy-dense foods, such as full-fat milk, white bread, full-fat spreads, and yogurts, provides growing children with carbohydrates, proteins, fatty acids, and vitamins and minerals. It is important to include enough essential fatty acids in a child's diet; these are vital for replenishing the fatty myelin insulation of nerves throughout the brain.

The anti-stroke diet

Stroke is a serious, damaging, and potentially fatal result of coronary artery disease—the clogging up of arteries. Eating for a healthy heart is the focus of most dietary and nutritional advice, with good reason. General guidelines recommend a diet containing foods low in fat and cholesterol; foods rich in fresh fruit and vegetables (for vitamins and plant-based phytochemicals); folate-rich foods or a supplement (reduces levels of homocysteine, a risk factor molecule for stroke); and whole grains. You also need to know which foods to avoid or restrict—especially those with a high fat or salt content.

EATING FOR INTELLIGENCE

Good nutrition can help you to maximize your intelligence. To a certain extent your mind power is genetically determined, but you can enhance nature's work with a little input of your own.

To prepare for a mental marathon, such as giving a speech or taking an exam, stock up on fresh fruit, such as apricots and strawberries, and dark-green leafy vegetables—seaweed is especially good. Cooked dried beans and peas, in a casserole, offer sustained energy and improve mental functioning. Seafood has brain-boosting properties. Serve a chargrilled tuna steak with noodles, baked salmon with lime, or a Caesar salad with anchovies. The chemicals in oily fish can enhance your memory and lift your mood.

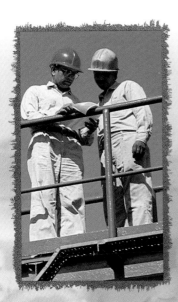

MID-AFTERNOON If there's more than about four hours between meals, a little snack is a good idea to refuel your brain and keep it functioning properly until the next pit stop—a few pretzels or a bag of nuts are great snack ideas.

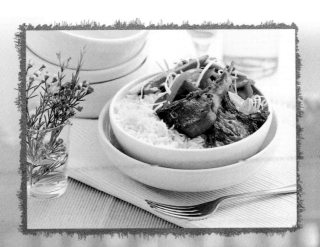

DINNER An evening meal is different from that of any other meal in the day: It improves logical reasoning and makes you feel more interested in what's going on around you. A modest carbohydrate-based meal is perfect.

BEDTIME SNACK If you feel hungry when you go to bed, you won't be able to sleep. A light carbohydrate-based snack such as a couple of crackers or a slice of bread and jam will allow your brain to relax and help you to drop off to sleep.

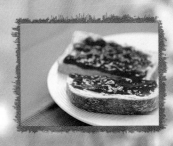

Food as brain medicine

The biochemistry of the brain is complex, but with some simple facts about how certain foods affect the brain, you can learn how to use food to positively influence how you feel and how you act.

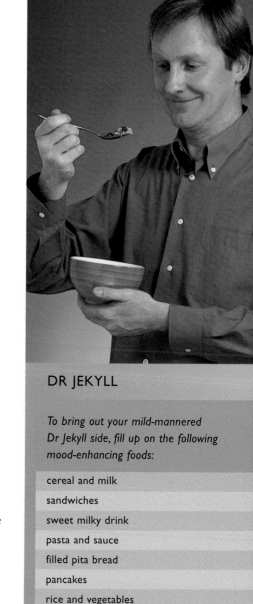

We have already outlined how you can maximize brain function by choosing particular foods at different times of the day to help suit your mind to different situations. Not only does food affect mental processes, it also affects emotional states of the mind and feelings of well-being.

NATURAL BRAIN CHEMICALS

Nerve cells in your brain and nervous system communicate via electrical and chemical messenger pathways; nerve signals travel along nerve fibers as electrical charges and between them as neurotransmitter chemicals. Some of these chemicals have an excitatory impact on nerve cells (promoting their activity) and others have an inhibitory effect (suppressing their activity). These biochemical factors affect your ability to make decisions, interact with others, and behave in a calm, rational manner. There are many types of these brain biochemicals, each with its own role to play: For example, acetylcholine is involved in learning and muscle

control; serotonin plays a role in mood regulation, eating, and sleeping; movement, attention, and learning are controlled by dopamine; and GABA (gamma-aminobutyric acid) is an inhibitory chemical involved in sleeping and eating.

GET THE "FEEL GOOD" FACTOR

How can food influence your brain? Here, we focus on the brain chemicals that you can influence through food—serotonin and dopamine.

Most neurotransmitters are made from constituents of the foods we eat. Serotonin, for example, requires a source of the essential amino acid tryptophan for its manufacture in the body. Once tryptophan-containing protein foods are digested, the tryptophan is transported to the brain in the bloodstream to make serotonin.

The brain is surrounded by a "molecular fence"—the blood–brain barrier—but tryptophan is allowed across. The more tryptophan that crosses this barrier, the more serotonin is produced. Tryptophan also needs glucose provided by carbohydrate foods, however, to help it cross this barrier. If you eat a high-protein, low-carbohydrate meal, you won't raise your serotonin levels as

DR JEKYLL

To bring out your mild-mannered Dr Jekyll side, fill up on the following mood-enhancing foods:

cereal and milk

sandwiches

sweet milky drink

pasta and sauce

filled pita bread

pancakes

rice and vegetables

filled jacket potato

effectively as with a low-protein, high-carbohydrate meal. So, to experience that "feel good" factor from a snack, rather than nibbling on a piece of cheese, make yourself a cheese sandwich with thick-cut bread.

Researchers have identified a link between serotonin levels and attention deficit hyperactivity disorder (ADHD) and Tourette's syndrome, a rare neurological disorder that causes physical and vocal tics. People with ADHD and Tourette's syndrome were found to

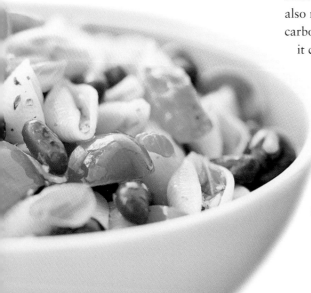

Mood-boosting pasta salad
A quick-to-prepare meal that will also give your brain a lift, a pasta salad combines carbohydrate with a low-protein content.

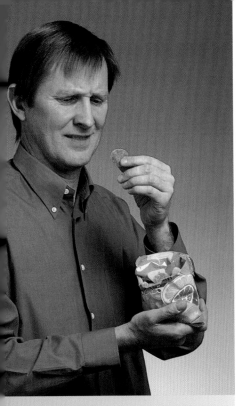

MR HYDE

If you're having a bad day, ask yourself whether you've been overindulging in the following bad mood foods:

package of cookies

several bars of chocolate

lots of strong coffee

lots of cups of tea

lots of sugary sweets

a big steak with no vegetables

lots of cheese

alcoholic drinks

have relatively low blood levels of tryptophan and serotonin.

Dopamine is another neurotransmitter made from tyrosine, an amino acid. High levels of dopamine can increase mental alertness and concentration. The amino acid tyrosine can be found in protein-rich foods. And this is just another reason why, to get the best for your brain and nervous system from the foods you eat, your diet should contain a good mixture of different nutrients.

EAT TO BEAT THE BLUES

Clinical syndromes such as depression or chronic anxiety are serious and distressing, but are luckily a far cry from the minor ups and downs and mood swings that affect almost all of us at one time or another. Whether your blues are brought on by an adverse reaction to shortening day length (known as seasonal affective disorder, or SAD) or just by general feelings of unrest, there are a few dietary tricks that may help you to break out of your negative frame of mind.

Don't be SAD

A common symptom of SAD, especially in women, is a craving for sugary, high-fat snacks, such as chocolate. Eating these sugary foods may actually help to relieve the recurrent depressive episodes associated with SAD by triggering insulin production. Insulin, in turn, releases glucose to accompany tryptophan across the blood–brain barrier, where it is converted to serotonin—the brain's natural mood elevator. But a sugary, carbohydrate-rich diet doesn't cure all SAD sufferers, and there is certainly no conclusive evidence to support these claims. In fact, some people will actually experience a greater feeling of depression after increasing their carbohydrate intake.

Fill up on folate

If you are feeling a bit low, you may not be getting the full quota of vitamins and minerals your body and brain need. A deficiency in folate (folic acid), for example, can lead to depression, irritability, and sleeplessness. Boosting your intake

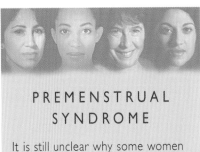

PREMENSTRUAL SYNDROME

It is still unclear why some women suffer from premenstrual syndrome (PMS). Symptoms include anxiety, irritability, poor concentration, and depression. One culprit is very high blood levels of estrogen in the days before a period. Vitamin B_6 helps to break down estrogen in the liver, so eating foods rich in B_6 (meat, fish, and whole grains) or taking a vitamin B_6 supplement can relieve symptoms in some women.

of this B vitamin through folate-rich foods such as spinach, broccoli, and oranges should help to raise your spirits, although a quicker fix would be to take a supplement—talk to your doctor about recommended dosages.

ADDITIVES AND BEHAVIOR— IS THERE A LINK?

Some psychological and behavioral problems have been linked to food additives, that is, any substance intentionally added to a food, be it to prevent food from spoiling or to enhance flavor or color. Additives may be naturally occurring or synthetic; a popular fallacy is that natural additives are safe whereas synthetic ones are potentially hazardous.

The concept that we have individual reactions to foods isn't new. The Roman poet Lucretius (96 to 55 B.C.) said "What is food to one

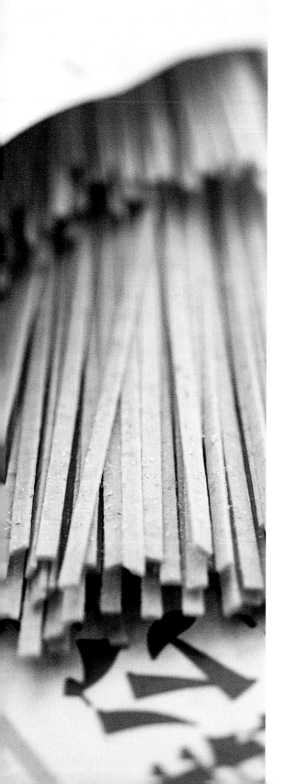

According to research, high-carbohydrate, low-protein foods such as jelly sandwiches, baked potatoes, and spaghetti with tomato sauce can help to combat stress.

man may be fierce poison to others," and research has concluded that diet can affect behavior of certain individuals, especially children. Initially, artificial colorings were the prime suspect in ADHD, but they are not always to blame. Hyperactivity is genetically determined, and certain foods can act as triggers. If you think that your child may have ADHD, you should seek professional help in modifying his or her diet.

EAT TO OVERCOME BRAIN HEALTH PROBLEMS

Use food positively to avoid certain conditions, such as migraine, and to prevent the neurological implications of others, such as adult-onset diabetes or Alzheimer's disease.

Migraine
The brain contains no pain receptors, so when you suffer a severe headache or migraine, although you may feel as though your brain is throbbing, it is actually the blood vessels outside the brain that are undergoing the discomfort. Although migraines are not always caused by food, some people can identify food-based triggers—cheese, chocolate, alcohol, and citrus fruits are the usual suspects. These foods contain vasodilating amines, which cause an adverse chemical reaction in some people as their livers try to break them down. This reaction causes changes in the blood vessels and membranes around the brain,

resulting in headache and migraine. If you suffer from migraines, keeping a food diary will help to identify any link between the headaches and diet.

Adult-onset diabetes
Also called non-insulin-dependent diabetes mellitus (NIDDM), adult-onset diabetes affects about 15 percent of people over the age of 50. If it is not controlled, the condition can cause the degeneration of the retina and nerves. It is most common in those who are overweight or of Asian origin. NIDDM can often be controlled by diet alone. Staying in a healthy weight range is advisable, and eating a diet high in complex carbohydrates with foods that contain soluble fiber, such as fruit, vegetables, and legumes, will help to keep this condition in check.

Alzheimer's disease
Most often a disease of the elderly, Alzheimer's is a steadily progressive type of dementia in which nerve cells degenerate, resulting in confusion, memory loss, and a lack of physical coordination. Although the media has reported the link between aluminium (from any dietary source or from cooking utensils) and Alzheimer's, researchers have yet to find conclusive evidence.

A common symptom of Alzheimer's disease is a loss of appetite. The vitamins C, E, B_{12}, B_6, folate, and beta-carotene have been associated with better performance in cognitive tests, so eat more foods with these vitamins or take a balanced supplement. There are also claims that coenzyme Q10, which is found in spinach, potatoes, yams, and soybeans, may be beneficial for Alzheimer's sufferers.

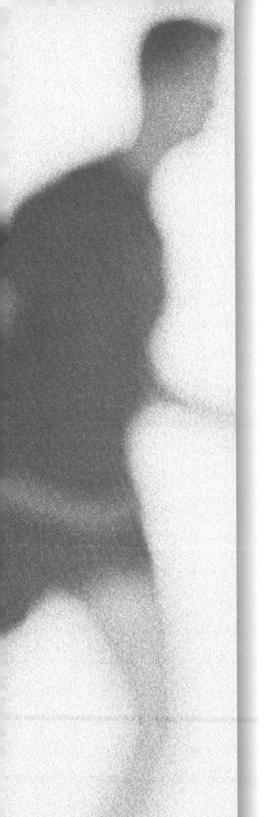

STIMULATE YOUR BRAIN

Your brain needs glucose and oxygen in order to operate. Some experts suggest that the lapses in memory and attention that become more frequent with aging may stem, in part, from compromised delivery of these basic fuels to the brain. So what can you do to make sure that your brain is getting the fuel it needs? Exercise—both physical and mental—is key. Working out your body and your mind is vital for a healthy brain to ward off the risk of stroke and to enhance your brain's already massive memory of skills and knowledge.

86 *Exercise is addictive. Find out how your brain can get hooked on the chemicals produced by a jog around the park or a game of tennis.*

88 *Discover how keeping your mind challenged and active, and improving memory skills, can help to combat age-related problems.*

Physical exercise for a healthy brain

You may often think about the benefits of exercise in terms of physical fitness, but have you ever considered activity to boost your mental power? Whatever your favorite sport, read on to find out how it can give your brain a workout.

Like other organs, your brain needs a constant supply of nutrients. In fact, your brain is a very fuel-hungry organ, requiring large amounts of glucose and oxygen to be delivered via the blood. Although your brain accounts for only 2 percent of your total body weight, it uses about 20 percent of the available glucose and oxygen—and you don't even have to be thinking hard!

A HEALTHY BODY MEANS A HEALTHY BRAIN

People who exercise have a healthy flow of blood to their vital organs, including the brain, because of their increased cardiovascular fitness. Studies have shown that rats exercised on a treadmill had higher levels of nerve growth factor, a chemical in the brain, than rats who were not exercised. Nerve growth factor promotes the development of neurons and encourages the connections between them that are vital in memory formation and information processing. So, as with rats, the fitter the person, the greater the capacity to increase the heart rate and so perform better mentally.

EXERCISE FOR INTELLIGENCE

So how fit is your brain? One of the best indicators of cardiovascular fitness is resting heart rate—the lower the better. Some professional athletes have a resting heart rate as low as 40 beats per minute, although a rate of between 60 and 80 beats per minute is the healthy norm for most people. Interestingly, people with a low resting heart rate tend to perform

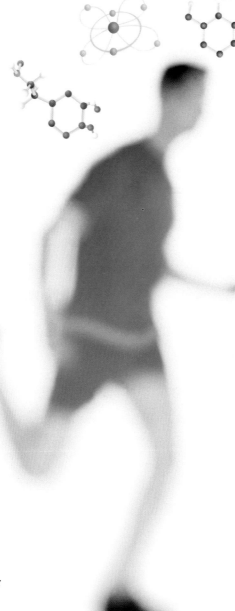

well on mentally taxing tasks such as the following serial sevens exercise:

- Sit quietly for a few minutes and measure your resting pulse (the easiest way is to count the number of heart beats in 15 seconds and multiply by 4). Make a note of this rate in beats per minute.
- Now subtract 7 from 978 and keep on subtracting 7. Say the numbers out loud and do it as fast and as accurately as you can.
- After two minutes of subtractions, take your pulse again. You should find that it has risen by 10 to 20 beats per minute.

Your brain is working harder and so needs a greater supply of glucose and oxygen, and your heart rate has responded to supply those needs. That isn't to say that fit people are better at math, just that the higher oxygen and glucose levels in their brains help them to cope with the added stress of the task.

JOGGER'S HIGH

In addition to affecting mental performance, exercise can benefit your mood. This is often thought to happen through the release of endorphins—the body's own opiates, which are known to be involved in processes such as painkilling and in our sensations of pleasure.

It is widely reported that exercise produces a feeling of euphoria—the so-called "jogger's high"—through

Chemical rush
Brain chemicals known as amines are produced during and after exercise, and these could account for the mood-boosting effects of physical exercise.

the production of endorphins, but there is little evidence to support this notion. In fact, in direct contradiction, one particular study reported a reduction in endorphin levels following exercise, despite an increased positive mood.

Amazing amines

Another set of brain chemicals are more likely to be the reason for the positive mood that usually follows exercise. These are the amines—norepinephrine, dopamine, and serotonin. Low levels of these natural brain chemicals are associated with depression, and there is evidence that exercise boosts their levels.

Blast the stress
A game of tennis is fast and furious—it gives you a real buzz. When through, you are physically exhausted, but the euphoric effects are unmistakable. It's a real stress buster.

STRESS BUSTING

Exercise is of particular benefit to people who are suffering from stress, depression, or anxiety, but it also seems to result in a more positive mood in psychologically healthy individuals. A single 30-minute period of exercise can reduce stress levels and feelings of depression and anxiety. It is the effect of regular exercise over a number of months, however, that has the most long-term beneficial

impact for mental health and an overall sense of well-being.

Regular exercise seems to have the effect of "immunizing" people against the stressful effects of everyday life—indeed it has been described as "stress inoculation." What's more, these beneficial effects are noticeable after only a few weeks in people who change from a sedentary lifestyle to one involving regular exercise.

EXERCISE ADDICTION

During exercise, heart rate increases, more oxygen is delivered to the brain, and the pupils dilate, rather like the "rush" experienced when illicit drugs are taken. The buzz of exercise can be addictive for some susceptible people. Some addicts of the amine rush will suffer from withdrawal symptoms, ranging from mild irritability to severe depression, if they can't get their exercise fix.

It is not just addiction to the amines associated with the jogger's high that cause the dependence, but a latching onto the feelings of well-being that surround exercise. However, like addiction to any other substance, exercise junkies often report that each time they exercise it takes them longer to feel the effects of jogger's high.

MEDITATIVE EXERCISES

Yoga and tai chi are both forms of physical exercise that involve an element of meditation, and therefore their impact on the brain is different from that of more vigorous sports. Meditation works upon the mind to alter the state of focused attention and heighten awareness. The mind is stimulated, although the rush of chemicals associated with aerobic

exercise is absent.

People who meditate regularly become adept at controlling their thoughts during meditation, which helps to eliminate emotional stresses.

ALONE OR ON A TEAM?

Some forms of exercise involve social interaction with friends, colleagues, or teammates. This social dimension is important to some people, but it cannot account for the positive effects of exercise on psychological health, which appear whether you play on a team or exercise alone. So in terms of brain health, you can take either a solitary jog in the park or play a game of football and you'll still get the same mental boost. On the other hand, group exercising may be an important factor in keeping you motivated and helping to

Mind bending
Keeping physically fit can help to keep you mentally fit. Any exercise with an aerobic component increases blood flow, and hence oxygen and glucose levels, to the brain.

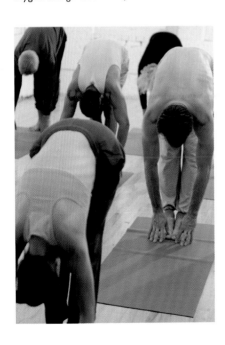

Exercise your mind

The cells and connections in your brain undergo changes over time. So what happens to your brain as you get older, and what can you do to ensure that your mind remains active, alert, and in the best mental shape?

Although your brain as an adult is, on average, four times bigger than when you were first born, this is largely due to an increase in the size of existing cells rather than the growth of new ones. The brain reorganizes itself during development, and neurons continue to make new connections with each other throughout life.

THE LEARNING PROCESS

During childhood, neurons within various brain structures mature and make connections at different times—an effect reflected by changes in a child's behavior. Generally, this is seen as increased control by the cerebral cortex and reflected by a movement toward more voluntary control of behavior. For example, a newborn baby may turn toward or grasp certain objects in a reflex manner. Within a few months this changes so that he or she can focus, reach out toward, and deliberately hold certain objects and can be soothed by familiar tones. These changes reflect the development of the brain regions responsible for hand–eye coordination and recognition of sounds.

Can any child be a genius?

Geniuses probably have lucky combinations of genes, but external factors play a part, too. Studies of rats have shown that those raised in a stimulating environment develop a thicker brain cortex and more neural connections than those raised in a bare cage. The extent to which these findings can be applied to humans is not clear—children do clearly benefit from a stimulating environment, but this will not turn them all into future Einsteins.

ASK THE EXPERT

The developing brain

At birth we have about 200 billion brain cells, called neurons. The number of neurons decreases throughout life, but the decline is gradual after the first year. In contrast, the number of connections—synapses—between neurons rises well into adulthood and declines slowly after the age of 70.

— Brain cells in billions
— Synapses in trillions

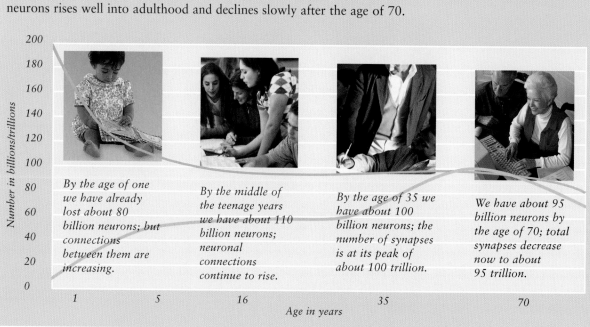

Number in billions/trillions

By the age of one we have already lost about 80 billion neurons; but connections between them are increasing.

By the middle of the teenage years we have about 110 billion neurons; neuronal connections continue to rise.

By the age of 35 we have about 100 billion neurons; the number of synapses is at its peak of about 100 trillion.

We have about 95 billion neurons by the age of 70; total synapses decrease now to about 95 trillion.

Age in years

REACHING MATURITY

The brain reaches its maximum size at the same time as the rest of the body—during adolescence. Then, during the teen years and sometimes into the early 20s, the brain shrinks to its fully mature size. The shrinkage is believed to be caused by the pruning of neural connections in the brain, to produce orderly pathways. Thereafter, in adulthood, the cortex of your brain loses over 100,000 neurons a day to cell death.

The idea that you have 100,000 fewer brain cells than you had yesterday, or up to 40 million fewer than at this time last year, sounds alarming. This loss, however, is negligible compared with the enormous number of cells that the brain contains. And neural connections are created every time you learn something new.

THE AGING BRAIN

By the age of 70 men will, on average, have lost about 10 percent of their brain volume; women lose slightly less. This tissue loss is not distributed equally throughout the brain—the frontal and temporal lobes appear to be more vulnerable to age-related loss of tissue.

How is this cell loss reflected by behavioral changes? As a general rule, older people tend to find it more difficult to learn new information and retrieve it from memory. This is characterised by the "tip-of-the-tongue" phenomenon—material is in the memory "store" but seems reluctant to be accessed. Older people also find it more difficult to react to novel stimuli than younger people. For example, they may find it more difficult to cope with an unexpected traffic situation.

GIVE YOUR BRAIN A WORKOUT

The motto for successful psychological aging is "use it or lose it." An 80-year-old who has completed crossword puzzles over a lifetime will be able to solve a new crossword puzzle as quickly as someone in his or her 20s. Each of the brain exercises shown here is designed to test different aspects of cognitive function, and if you do them a few times a week you should see a rapid improvement in your brain fitness.

Give the different letters of the alphabet the numerical values 1 to 26 (A = 1, B = 2, etc.). Try to think of words in which the sum of the letters adds up to 40. Next time you can use a different figure.

Turn a book or a newspaper upside down. Read the page from the bottom to the top. Notice how much more effort is needed to make sense of the structure of sentences.

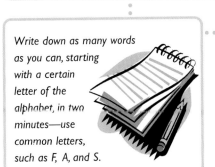

Delve into your memory and try to recall the names of teachers or fellow pupils in your class at school. See if you can remember details such as what they wore or what kind of person they were. Next time, think about a past workplace or a street where you once lived. You will be surprised at how much you haven't forgotten!

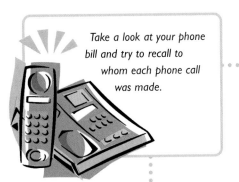

Write down as many words as you can, starting with a certain letter of the alphabet, in two minutes—use common letters, such as F, A, and S.

Concentrate on the second hand of a watch or clock for one minute. Now close your eyes and see if you can time a minute exactly.

Take a look at your phone bill and try to recall to whom each phone call was made.

If you have access to a computer, turn the mouse round, so that moving the ball left and up makes the cursor move right and down.

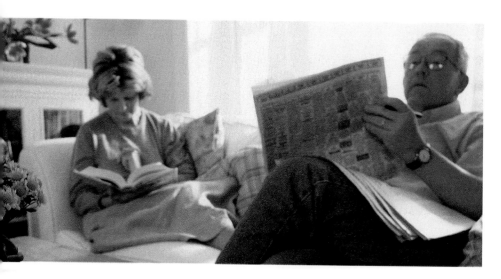

The power of reading
To improve the amount you can recall, try thinking through what you have just read when you put down your book or paper.

There is enormous individual variability in the extent to which older people fall prey to such changes; some people appear to be relatively immune to them.

THE DEMENTIAS

At the extreme end of aging-related cognitive decline lie the dementias. Age is the most important risk factor for dementia—the number of individuals with Alzheimer's disease, for example, doubles every five years in the elderly population.

Alzheimer's disease is the most common of the dementias; other causes of dementia are cerebro-vascular disease, Pick's disease, and Creutzfeldt–Jakob disease (CJD). The brain of an Alzheimer's sufferer is characterised by marked cerebral atrophy—the brain appears to have "withered" in the skull. This atrophy occurs as a result of reduced levels of the neurotransmitter acetylcholine and the appearance of plaques and

tangles in the neuronal circuits. These plaques and tangles are abnormal microscopic structures that are believed to "unwire" the neural circuits responsible for storage and processing of information in the brain. There is some evidence that there is a genetic predisposition for dementia, but this is clearly not the whole story—many individuals who have the appropriate genetic makeup for the disease do not develop it.

Protective exercise

People who are mentally active are to some extent protected from Alzheimer's—if they develop the disorder at all it tends to be later in life and progresses at a slower rate. It seems that such individuals build up a "cognitive reserve" that they can tap into when their own mental resources become worn away. It is not known exactly how this works but it seems that there is a sub-population of neurons that continues to grow and make connections while others are being lost. If this special subset of neurons is encouraged to bloom through mental stimulation it may help to delay a certain amount of cognitive decline.

MAKING MEMORIES

Our brains are full of memories, but where are they all stored? The hippocampus plays an important role—people with damage to this part of the brain cannot form new mem-ories. But anything learned before the damage is unaffected, suggesting that memories are stored elsewhere.

Intriguingly, people who have damage to the hippocampus can learn new skills. If repeatedly presented with the same puzzle, they can solve it more quickly each time, although they do not have any memory of learning it.

Well connected

At the microscopic level, information is stored in the brain using neural circuits; that is, it is stored via the activity of a vast network of interconnected neurons. Memory formation involves the strengthening of the connections between these neurons. This process involves increasing the number of effective synaptic connections between neurons by shifting the location of synapses so that the input has more effect on its target neuron.

Short- and long-term memory

One useful way of thinking about memory is as a store of information. Nearly all data is first kept in a temporary store called short-term memory. In order to be remembered later, it has to enter a long-term store—a process called consolidation. Once there, material can be accessed more or less at will.

MAXIMIZE YOUR MEMORY

A good memory is a powerful tool. Different strategies seem to help different people to strengthen their memory capacity, but there are a few basic techniques you can try.

- **Rehearse your lines** By repeating, for example, a telephone number over and over again, you can help the information transfer from short-term to long-term memory.
- **Go multimodal** If you have a list of names to remember, say them out loud, listen carefully to the sound of the words as you say them, write them down, and focus on how the words look as you do so. This combination may help to get the information into the memory store.
- **Draw a map** A mindmap is a representation of information in a picture, where different aspects of the topic or concept are connected on a diagram. Studying the mindmap will help you to recall the information later.

Another exercise that some people find helpful is to tell themselves a story—this can be a valuable way to store and retrieve information, a technique called the "method of loci."

With this method you need to first picture a familiar route such as the path you take from your front door into one room of your house. Now picture 10 locations along the route, for example, it might be your doormat, a telephone table, a painting on the wall, the bottom of the stairs, and the lamp on the landing. Take some time to rehearse these locations so that you can easily remember them in the right order.

Now add images to these locations to help you remember all the things you have to do today. For example:

- **Feed the dog** Visualize your dog lying on the doormat.
- **Remember to pay the electricity bill** Picture your telephone table being struck by a bolt of lightning.
- **Meet a friend for lunch** Visualize your friend in the painting.
- **Go to the supermarket** Imagine yourself tripping over bags of groceries sitting at the foot of your stairs.
- **Return your library books** Picture the lampshade as glowing pages of a book.

You should be able to remember each thing accurately and in order. The more vivid the images, the more likely are they to stick in your mind. With practice, you will be able to replace old items with new ones and to extend your journey so that you can use the method to remember more and more.

BOOST YOUR MENTAL CAPACITY

In addition to using the activities in this book, keep your mind active by using problem-solving puzzles and crosswords. Many card games are excellent at stimulating memory and concentration. Computer games also involve these skills and are excellent at keeping reaction times fast. Keep yourself well informed and socialize to discuss current issues with friends and family.

Go on-line There is a wealth of information available via new technologies such as the Internet. Surfing the Net can be educational and challenging. Some older people find it difficult to get started using such technologies, but once they do, most find it stimulating and enjoyable.

There are many evening classes and starter packages around with good support, as well as books and videos that guide you through getting onto and using the Internet. The breadth of topics is ever widening—travel, health, news are but a few; tapping into this resource can help to keep your knowledge and computer skills up to date.

Mapping your route
When planning an event, such as a vacation, make a mindmap to help you to remember everything you have to do. In this case, thinking of beachwear prompts you to think of sunscreen, and so on.

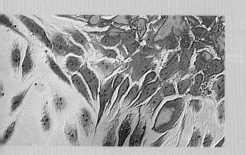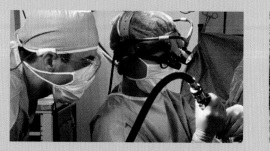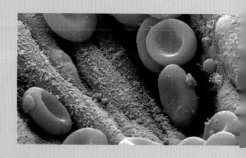

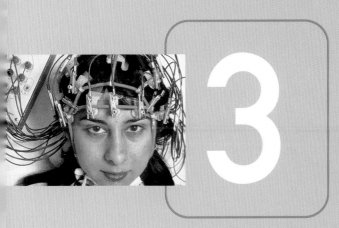

3

What happens
when things go wrong

Knowing what can go wrong

We have all experienced the occasional headache, which disappears without consequence. Serious neurological conditions are rare, although with some, such as Alzheimer's disease and stroke, the incidence increases with age.

AGING PROCESSES

An adult's brain contains around 100 billion neurons or nerve cells. Each of us is born with twice that number—all the neurons we will ever have. In our first year of life there is massive rewiring in the brain, and up to half of our original brain cells die as we develop and learn to move and speak. From this time on, there is a gradual loss of cells—a mere 100,000 a day—as a consequence of neurons specializing in order to function more efficiently. The nervous system is

MORE COMMON

HEADACHE	SHINGLES
An estimated 45 million Americans experience chronic headaches.	Ten percent of normal adults, most over the age of 50, will get shingles in their lifetimes.
This is the most commonly encountered neurological symptom.	The shingles virus affects vital nerves at the top of the spinal cord.

remarkably flexible: It can compensate for some of this age-related loss of neurons by increasing the connections between remaining cells, and some parts of the brain can even take on the roles of others. Quite a large amount of nervous tissue can be lost before there are any noticeable signs or symptoms.

As we get older, we expect that at some stage we will have to wear reading glasses to correct focusing problems (presbyopia) or possibly that we will have some difficulty hearing (presbycusis): Both are gradually developing neurological conditions. Other age-related conditions are less easy to accept: The risk of contracting certain diseases that result from massive brain cell loss, such as Alzheimer's disease, do increase with age, but these conditions will not affect everyone; there are other influences to be taken into consideration.

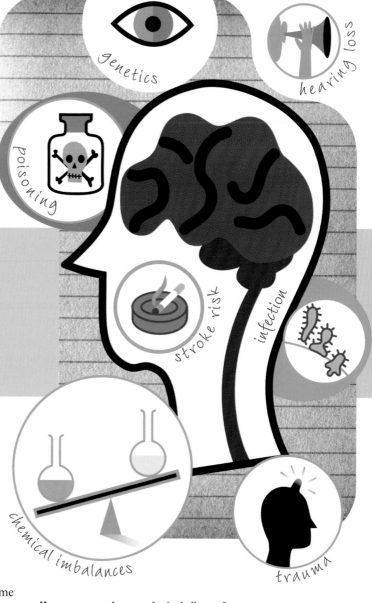

How common is neurological disease?
The incidence in the United States of selected neurological conditions are shown in the colored band above. Figures relate either to the number of new cases reported in a year or to number in the population affected (U.S. 2002 population = 287 million). Although the chart shows the average risk of being affected, when considering other factors and the potential causes of neurological diseases, the risk for specific individuals will vary.

PHYSICAL INJURY—TRAUMA

The rigid bony "containers" of the skull and spine protect the vulnerable, delicate tissues of the central nervous system against harm and physical injury in all but the most extreme circumstances. A blow to the head can cause a range of injury from mild concussion to severe brain damage and even death. In the U.S., each year there are more than 50,000 head injuries severe enough to cause deaths. Traffic accidents, firearm-related assaults, falls, and sporting injuries are the main causes. Most people with a head injury make a full recovery, but about 1,500 people each year are left with a permanent brain injury. A similar number damage their spinal cord, usually in the vulnerable neck region, which leads to paralysis below the level of the injury; whether or not paralysis is permanent depends on the degree and site of the injury.

are rare, although these are more likely in a child if the parents are related. One inherited condition is Tay–Sachs disease, which mainly affects Ashkenazi Jews and French Canadians. Both parents can pass on the gene to their offspring. Genetic screening is now available to help reduce the incidence of this disease. Other familial conditions are heart disease and stroke. Data on the frequency of common diseases in the population suggests that illnesses such as Alzheimer's and Parkinson's disease have a genetic link, but this is not yet clearly proven.

DEGENERATIVE DISORDERS

There are a number of slowly progressive diseases that may affect the whole brain or areas of the brain due to excessive death of brain cells; precisely why this happens is unknown. The most common example is Alzheimer's disease; it seems that some people are genetically

LESS COMMON

STROKE	DEMENTIAS	EPILEPSY	MULTIPLE SCLEROSIS
600,000 per year (160,000 deaths)	4 million people are affected by Alzheimer's disease, the most prevalent of the dementias (50 to 70 percent of all cases). Vascular dementia is the second most common form found in the U.S. population.	2.3 million people are affected.	350,000 to 500,000 people are afflicted.
		PARKINSON'S DISEASE 1 million people	**MOTOR NEURON DISEASE** 5 to 10 per 100,000
		MENINGITIS 5–10 per 100,000	
		TUMORS (malignant and benign) 18 per 100,000 (1 in 5,555)	

CARDIOVASCULAR DISEASE AND STROKE

Stroke is the third most common cause of death in the Western world; most are due to a blockage of the brain circulation by a blood clot, and the rest are due to brain hemorrhage. The main risk factors for stroke are smoking, high blood pressure, and diabetes mellitus. People with other circulatory disease (such as coronary artery disease or angina) or a family history of stroke are also at higher risk. The risk of stroke increases with age, reflecting the fact that high blood pressure, diabetes, and heart disease also rise with age.

GENETICS AND HEREDITARY FACTORS

Genes are the blueprints for our body chemistry and structure, and the genes we inherit from our parents can predispose us to disease. Inherited neurological diseases

predisposed to developing the disease, but the precise genetic factors are not known. In another well-known example, Parkinson's disease, there is a localized loss of brain cells—in the basal ganglia—resulting in the characteristic tremors and loss of muscle control.

INFECTION

Infection of the nervous system is relatively rare but can be very serious. The most feared infection is meningitis, but disease-causing organisms don't only attack the meningeal membranes; they also crucially target the brain tissue itself in encephalitis as well as the spinal cord in myelitis. Part of the mystery of meningitis is why the bacterium commonly responsible for the infection—the *Meningococcus*—can be carried harmlessly in the throats of some people but not others. Most viruses or bacteria that cause disease travel to the brain or spinal cord in the bloodstream, but they can also move to the brain from nearby sites of infection, such as an ear or sinus, although this is extremely rare.

Abnormal malignant cells
This mass of cancerous cells is dispersing after becoming detached from a tumor. Such cells often settle at sites within the brain to form secondary tumors.

TUMORS

As elsewhere in the body, tumors of the central nervous system can be either benign (noncancerous) or malignant (cancer forming). But because of the delicacy of brain tissue, a benign tumor can be as damaging as a malignant one. Secondary tumors—metastases—from cancer in another organ, such as the lung, often spread to the brain. The most common primary tumors are gliomas—cancer of the glial cells— which are more common in young adulthood. Meningiomas, which are benign and slow-growing tumors of the meninges, compress neural tissues rather than invading them like other cancers, and commonly affect people over 55, often without any symptoms.

PSYCHOLOGICAL DISTURBANCES WITH A BIOCHEMICAL BASIS

Some psychological conditions arise through behavioral or mood factors, but here we concentrate on those with an underlying biochemical—neurophysiological—basis. Some symptoms previously thought to have a psychological cause are now known to be the result of a physical imbalance of chemicals within the brain. Depression, the most common psychological disturbance, carries a wide range of symptoms, from mild blues, which may affect most people to some degree in their lives, to psychotic delusional despair. Severe depression requiring medical treatment is associated with reduced serotonin levels in the brain's limbic system. Schizophrenia is rarer and is thought to be caused by abnormalities of dopamine metabolism in the brain. These imbalances result in altered thought processing and personality destruction, most commonly in young adults.

NUTRITIONAL DEFICIENCIES

Many nutrients in food are essential to the health of the nervous system. Dietary deficiencies are common worldwide, but they are rare in the West. When they do occur, they are usually due to digestive abnormalities caused by conditions such as alcoholism. Deficiency of vitamin B_1 is probably the most common deficiency that can cause neurological disease and is frequently seen in alcoholics. Also, vitamin B_{12} deficiency can lead to pernicious anemia as well as neural damage, resulting in confusion, general weakness, and numbness or tingling in limbs; it is most common in people over 50 because the stomach's ability to absorb B_{12} decreases with age.

POISONING

Many substances ingested accidentally or deliberately are toxic to the nervous system; the most common of these is alcohol. Long-term abuse of alcohol—alcoholism—leads to depression of various mental functions; in contrast, an overdose of alcohol (for example half a bottle of whisky on an empty stomach) can lead to alcohol poisoning, possibly resulting in coma, convulsions, and death. Carbon monoxide causes more than 5,000 deaths in the United States per year. More than half of these occur in automobiles. Carbon monoxide binds to red blood cells, preventing them from carrying life-supporting oxygen: Essentially it starves the nervous system of oxygen, and brain cell death occurs. Lead poisoning can also cause nerve damage, although it is less common now that lead-based paints are no longer used.

IT'S NOT TRUE!

"Depression is all in the mind"

Depression is not a disease of the brain alone. Most people with depression experience real physical symptoms, such as muscle weakness and loss of energy. Sometimes a person experiences pains and heaviness in the chest, which could be mistaken for heart problems, or aches in the limbs. Often someone with depression has a greatly reduced appetite and suffers from constipation. The quality of sleep is poor and sufferers typically awake early in the morning.

Who's who—brain and nervous system experts

Which health professional you meet and when depends on the neurological symptoms you experience. From physical to psychological, each specialty has its own expertise, though you will find overlap among them.

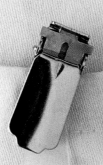

NEUROSURGEON

Working closely with neurologists, neurosurgeons are trained to deal with conditions that can be treated surgically, such as spinal cord compression, tumors of the nervous system, and subarachnoid hemorrhage. A patient would be referred by a general practitioner or neurologist. Neurosurgical departments depend on specialist intensive care support after an operation and so are almost always located in specialist centers only.

RADIOLOGIST

This hospital specialist is expert in the diagnosis of disease from medical images. Neurology is one specialty that relies on radiology for accurate diagnostic support, because the brain and spinal cord are hidden within protective casings. As well as deciding how much radiation a particular imaging procedure requires, a radiologist examines the data (be they X-ray film or digital scans) and writes a report for the referring doctor on the likely diagnosis.

PSYCHIATRIST

Psychiatry is one of the largest medical specialties, in both hospitals and the community. A psychiatrist has trained in the diagnosis and management of disorders of mood, behavior, thought, and addiction. Such disorders can be caused by a primary neurochemical disturbance or may be a symptom of a disease being dealt with by a neurologist. Psychiatrists provide services from counseling to drug therapy and electroconvulsive therapy.

CLINICAL PSYCHOLOGIST

Not usually medically qualified, a clinical psychologist has extensive training plus specialist clinical experience. Clinical psychologists base their practice on theories of behavior and thinking processes rather than chemical imbalances. They are involved in assessing the diverse aspects of higher mental functions, as well as giving psychotherapy and counseling.

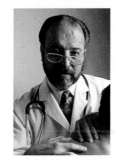

NEUROLOGIST

Neurologists are medical specialists with expertise in the diagnosis and treatment of diseases of the nervous system. All neurologists deal with disorders that can be treated without surgery, such as multiple sclerosis, Parkinson's disease, epilepsy, headache, and stroke. Neurologists may be hospital based or work in the community. They often work closely with physical and occupational therapists.

DEVELOPMENTAL PSYCHOLOGIST

Although they have a similar background to clinical psychologists, developmental psychologists have a specialist interest in the growth and development of the human mind in children with cerebral palsy, autism, Aspergers syndrome, and other specific learning handicaps. They work in close liaison with occupational therapists and physical therapists, together with either a pediatrician or a pediatric neurologist.

GERIATRIC NURSE

This covers a multitude of professionals, from the fully trained hospital nurse caring for an elderly patient admitted to hospital in an emergency, to the nursing assistant at a nursing home. A geriatric nurse may be involved in rehabilitating victims of stroke, looking after patients with dementia, or helping people who are frail but otherwise healthy; the range of abilities and training varies accordingly from job to job.

FINDING OUT WHAT IS WRONG

The first port of call when a person experiences any neurological symptoms is usually a general practitioner (GP) or internist. After assessing the problem, this doctor may decide to refer the person to a neurologist.

It is reassuring to know that doctors have a whole host of diagnostic tools at their disposal. These range from simple blood tests performed in the hospital laboratories to high-tech digital imaging, such as MRI scanning, to the standard technique of EEG, which measures brain activity. Which investigative tests, if any, a person undergoes will depend on the outcome of the first consultation with the neurologist. The results of any diagnostic procedures and tests are gathered together by the neurologist to determine the cause of a problem. These pieces of the "illness jigsaw" may not always fit easily into the classic textbook picture, so a patient should not be too concerned if a diagnosis takes some time.

Medical history and examination

The first visit starts with a discussion about the neurological symptoms, followed by a physical examination and specific tests to assess brain and nervous system function.

HISTORY—A TWO-WAY CONVERSATION

Of all medical specialties, neurology—the diagnosis and treatment of nervous disorders—is the most dependent on a medical history and the least able to rely upon other confirmatory tests, such as laboratory tests and imaging. A comfortable and communicative relationship between doctor and patient is, therefore, vital to the diagnostic process. To find out what is wrong, the neurologist will encourage a person to tell his or her own story, known as "taking a history," and ask questions about symptoms, past health, any conditions that run in the family, and information about work and social situations.

General information about symptoms

The doctor may first wish to know whether you are right- or left-handed, as the brain has different functions in right and left hemispheres, which may be partly determined by your dominant hand. The next questions are typically open-ended to allow a full description of the symptoms, which could range from headaches, blackouts, and changes in muscle strength or sensation to loss of coordination, tremulousness, loss of vision, poor memory, and difficulty in controlling the bladder and bowel. Once the general picture is established, the doctor focuses on individual symptoms and asks specific questions to gain a better understanding.

Symptom specifics

Key questions are, "When did a symptom begin?" and "How has it changed over time?" Some illnesses, such as Parkinson's disease, produce slow but progressive degeneration, but others, such as a stroke, may happen suddenly. Extra details about associated symptoms may help to distinguish one illness from another. Headaches are a good example: The pain of a migraine is classically felt more on one side of the head, has a throbbing intensity with an associated sensitivity to light and noise, and is accompanied by intense nausea; migraines may be preceded by flashing lights or auras. In contrast, a tension headache feels like a band of pressure around the head, with a squeezing sensation; it may also be linked to low mood or anxiety. Associated symptoms may help to determine the cause of a blackout: Fainting is typically preceded by dizziness and sweating, whereas an epileptic seizure may be preceded by an "aura," such as a peculiar smell, hallucination, or déjà vu.

Past medical information

An individual's medical history is of great importance. As well as finding out about any chronic disease, such as diabetes or high blood pressure, the doctor will want to know of any incidence of other neurological illness. Multiple sclerosis, for instance, can be diagnosed only if there has been more than one episode affecting different parts of the nervous system on different occasions. The doctor will also ask about long-term medications, now or in the past, and drug allergies.

Family medical history

Some conditions run in families, so the doctor will ask if any close family members have suffered from neurological complaints. Ask brothers, sisters, parents, grandparents, and other relatives to see if anyone has been affected.

Social situation

The doctor will ask about work and social circumstances; this information is valuable when deciding on rehabilitation, aids, and insurance benefit eligibility. Some conditions, such as epilepsy, will have implications for driving, which may impact work or home life. The doctor will also ask about alcohol consumption, smoking, and illicit drug use.

HELP YOUR DOCTOR TO HELP YOU

Making the most of a visit

If you or someone you know needs to consult a doctor about neurological symptoms, bear in mind that although symptoms are common, serious neurological disease is rare. Also, remember that your doctor is not a mindreader— you hold all the vital information. Be prepared to answer the following questions.

- *When did your symptoms start?*
- *Are they getting worse?*
- *Do they come and go, or are they constant?*
- *Have you had them before?*
- *Has any family member had this complaint?*

Take an eye witness—If you have experienced a loss of consciousness, it will help the doctor to speak to someone who saw the episode happen.

Take a photo—some neurological conditions result in a change in appearance. An old photograph can be useful, particularly if your doctor didn't know you well beforehand.

Try to learn about your condition and don't be afraid to ask questions; take a notepad to visits to help you remember important facts.

Bright or flashing lights?
Tell your doctor if you experience any adverse sensitivity to light—photophobia.

Painful eye?
If your eye becomes suddenly painful and red, go straight to the doctor or hospital.

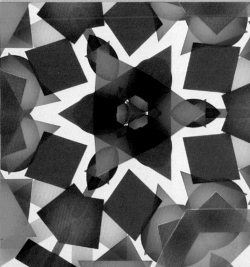

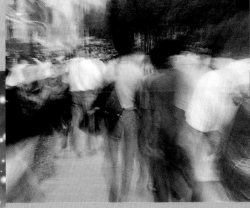

Blurred or tunnel vision?
If your vision becomes blurred or you experience tunnel vision, consult your doctor immediately.

THE PHYSICAL EXAMINATION

The process of examination begins before most people are aware of it. Key information can be gleaned by the doctor just from observing a person entering the room, and any problems with speech, mood, or memory are usually apparent when answering questions.

the reflexes may be less apparent or even absent. The Babinski reflex is tested by scratching the outside edge of the sole of the foot. In a healthy person, the big toe curls towards the scratch—a Babinski-negative response. If the toe curls upward and away—a Babinski-positive response—it suggests a disease of the nervous system.

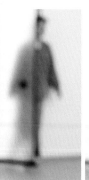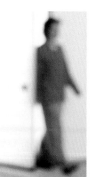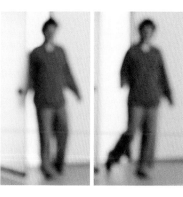

A doctor can learn a lot about the nervous system by watching the way a person walks. For example, people with disease of the cerebellum may compensate for a loss of balance by widely spacing their feet.

Testing sight, hearing, and balance

To assess vision, a neurologist uses a letter chart similar to that used by an optician. Other sight tests include
- Checking visual fields by assessing the ability to see a small object, such as a pen, out of the corner of the eye
- Testing color vision using a special series of camouflaged numbers known as Ishihara charts
- Examining the back of the eye (the retina) with a handheld instrument that shines a light into the eye
- Checking the range and control of eye movements and noting any double vision

Such checks give the doctor vital information, in particular whether there is evidence of raised pressure within the skull or previous inflammation of the optic nerve.

The doctor assesses hearing using a tuning fork. To detect whether both ears have the same hearing level, a vibrating tuning fork is held overhead and the person indicates whether the sound is equally loud in both ears.

The balance organs of the brain and inner ear can be tested when you move from a sitting to a lying position; the doctor looks for a sideways flickering of the eye.

Checking reflexes

A doctor checks a reflex, for example the knee jerk, by using a tendon hammer; a faster or slower, or stronger or weaker response could indicate a problem. If central nerve pathways are damaged, such as following a stroke or onset of multiple sclerosis, reflexes become stronger and quicker; if peripheral nerves are impaired, as in polio,

Measuring muscle power

The doctor assesses the symmetry of the limbs, watching for any tremor. The strength of the limbs is tested by gently pushing against movements the patient is asked to make. Different patterns of muscle weakness may be characteristic of particular diseases.

Testing sensation and coordination

The doctor tests sensation using a variety of stimuli—a pin, cotton wool, vibration (from a tuning fork)—and notes whether or not each one can be felt. To test coordination, the doctor may ask you to alternately touch your nose and then his or her fingertips.

Testing higher brain functions

The examination of the complex brain tasks performed by the cerebral cortex includes
- **Language skills** The doctor will listen to how fluent and articulate the person's conversation is.
- **Memory and recall** Questions are asked on the time of day and the person's current location, and simple tests of repetition and recall (using three objects) are conducted.
- **Mathematical ability** A typical example is being asked to subtract 7 repeatedly from 100 for two minutes.
- **Object recognition** Objects could be auditory, tactile (drawing a number in the palm of the hand), or 3-D.

Higher brain function can be measured numerically using psychometric tests, which are usually performed under the supervision of a neuropsychologist.

Laboratory tests

What happens to blood or cerebrospinal fluid once the sample is taken? Doctors use a range of tests to find vital clues to the cause of the neurological complaint.

TESTS ON BLOOD

Giving a sample of blood from a vein in the arm can be slightly uncomfortable, but it is over in a minute or two. Even if more than one blood test has been ordered, several tubes can be filled, in turn, from one needle prick. Once in self-sealed tubes, the blood is whisked off to the laboratory for detailed analysis. Half of the volume of blood is made up of blood cells, and the remaining half is a straw-colored fluid—plasma. Proteins, sugars, and minerals all circulate around the body dissolved within the plasma.

Counting cells

There are three types of blood cells—red cells, white cells, and platelets. Red blood cells are filled with hemoglobin, a protein that carries oxygen around the body; white blood cells fight infection; and tiny platelets form blood clots. A full blood count estimates the numbers of each blood cell and is performed by an automated machine.

In addition to counting the number of red blood cells, the machine also measures the amount of hemoglobin they contain. By using information about the hemoglobin content and the number of red blood cells, the machine can estimate cell size. If a patient is anemic, for example, the doctor will be particularly interested in the size of the red blood cells. Large red cells are a hallmark of vitamin B_{12} deficiency, which could indicate the more serious condition of pernicious anemia.

Various types of white blood cell—lymphocytes, neutrophils, and eosinophils—are important in the diagnosis of neurological complaints. Reduced lymphocytes may be a marker of HIV infection, which may be associated with dementia, neuropathy, opportunistic infections of the brain, and tumors.

Elevated levels of any blood cells can have many causes, including bone marrow diseases such as leukemia. In leukemia, large numbers of immature cells are produced, which can increase the "stickiness" of blood and reduce its ability to flow through the blood vessels of the brain, thereby predisposing the sufferer to stroke and thrombosis of the cerebral veins.

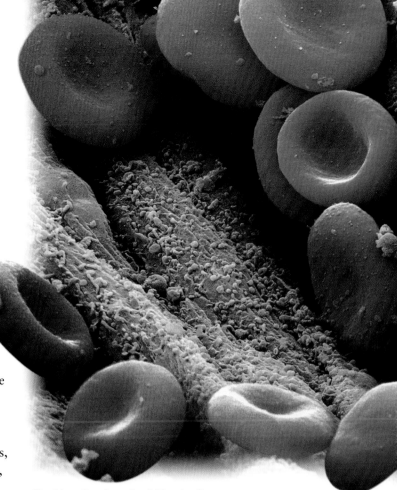

Checking the size of red blood cells
Overlarge red blood cells—called macrocytes—are indicative of vitamin B_{12} deficiency, which can cause spinal cord degeneration as well as damage to peripheral nerves and the optic nerve.

Measuring clotting ability

The clotting system of the blood contains many different interacting chemicals that are dissolved in the plasma and operate in a cascade, once activated. The tendency to form blood clots is counterbalanced by a system to break them down. Certain inherited conditions increase the tendency of the blood to clot and are associated with a higher risk of stroke; abnormal clotting may also be associated with migraines and recurrent stroke.

Analyzing minerals

Minerals such as sodium and calcium dissolved in the plasma are called electrolytes. The relative concentrations of electrolytes are some of the first test results the doctor will want to see. A low sodium level or a high calcium level may be associated with confusion and drowsiness, whereas low levels of both sodium and calcium may increase the risk of an epileptic seizure. Disorders of kidney and liver function are associated with increases in toxic metabolites in the blood, which

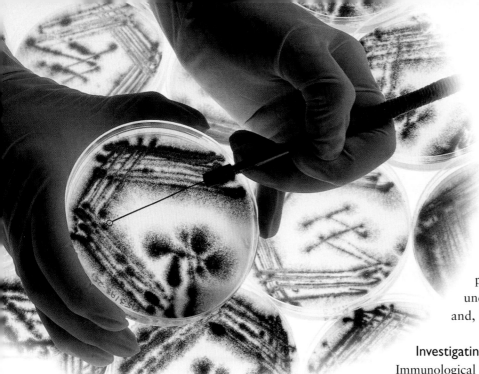

and may cause depression and even psychosis. Long-term thyroid underactivity damages the cerebellum and, if severe, can lead to a coma.

can disturb the brain's regulation and result in coma. Low magnesium levels can cause seizures, and reduced blood levels of potassium could cause muscle cramps and weakness.

Checking blood glucose

Swings in blood glucose levels have visible effects on the functioning of the central nervous system: High levels can cause nerve damage (neuropathy), whereas low levels can cause confusion. High blood glucose levels indicate that a person has diabetes mellitus, a major risk factor for stroke. Excessively high glucose levels can also cause a complex metabolic derangement (diabetic ketoacidosis) in people with insulin-dependent diabetes or a state of overly concentrated and highly "sticky" blood in those with non-insulin-dependent (adult-onset) diabetes.

Checking hormone levels

Hormones are another set of chemicals present in the plasma. The most commonly tested is thyroid-stimulating hormone (TSH). An overactive thyroid gland may be associated with tremulousness and agitation, and sometimes with a disease of the muscles that move the eye. Underactivity is also problematic

The shingles virus
Laboratory tests can identify the microbial cause of a neurological complaint—a possible cause is herpes zoster, the virus that causes shingles.

Investigating infection

Immunological tests examine the body's defense mechanisms and the most common test looks at the antibodies circulating in the plasma. The presence of antibodies suggests exposure to a particular infection, and sometimes the type of antibody gives information about whether the infection is current or occurred in the past; similar tests are carried out on cerebrospinal fluid.

Different antibodies are produced in response to different stimuli; sometimes they may even be targeted against body tissues—so-called autoantibodies. Antibodies that are toxic to the nervous system may be produced in conditions such as cancer. Other nerve-specific antibodies can cause disease: In the condition myasthenia gravis, antibodies block acetylcholine receptors and so impair communication between muscles and nerves, resulting in weak muscles that tire easily.

Antibody tests are used to establish the presence of antibodies to determine whether an infection is caused by viruses (such as HIV), bacteria (such as *Meningococcus*), protozoa (such as *Toxoplasma*), or fungi (such as *Cryptococcus*). A laboratory technician then uses special stains to highlight the offending pathogen and analyzes the sample under a microscope to identify possible causes. Even if analysis reveals no infecting organisms, some of the specimen will be put onto a culture medium to see if any bacteria grow; at the same

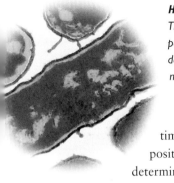

***Haemophilus influenzae* bacteria**
This germ is just one of the many pathogens that can cause potentially dangerous inflammation of the meningeal membranes—meningitis.

time, antibiotic disks are positioned on the Petri dish to determine which particular ones the germs are sensitive to.

TESTS ON CEREBROSPINAL FLUID

The cerebrospinal fluid (CSF) bathes the entire central nervous system. To gain access to this fluid, a doctor performs what is called a spinal tap using a special needle to make a tiny hole in the lumbar, or lower, part of the spinal canal in order to withdraw 1 to 2 teaspoonsful of fluid. Laboratory analysis of CSF can help to detect any inflammation or infection of the brain tissue or the spinal cord, such as meningitis or myelitis.

Looking for inflammation or infection

Healthy CSF is clear and colorless; in someone with an infection of the nervous system, such as meningitis, the fluid may be cloudy and white. The most important test to confirm an infection is to examine the sample of fluid under a microscope. In cases of bacterial meningitis, for example, the bacteria may be visible after the CSF sample is treated with a special stain—although the organisms are not always present. Another microscopic test involves counting white blood cells: There should be fewer than five white cells per cubic millimeter—if levels are higher, there is inflammation or infection. The type of white cell present can determine whether the infection is bacterial or viral.

Any bleeding into the CSF, as in a subarachnoid hemorrhage, is indicated by a dramatic rise in the number of red blood cells. A test can be carried out to check for the presence of hemoglobin or its breakdown products, which will give the doctor vital clues about whether or not there is bleeding.

Checking protein and sugar levels

Normally, the protein content of CSF is much lower than that of blood. A rise in protein levels could indicate increased blood vessel leakage, either because of inflammation or because of abnormal blood vessels (such as those in a tumor). In some conditions, such as multiple sclerosis, the presence of an immunoglobulin protein, can support a diagnosis of the illness. A great reduction in the sugar content of the CSF could indicate bacterial meningitis.

HAVING A SPINAL TAP

The doctor told me exactly what he was going to do and that it was a simple and straightforward test.

I had to get into a robe and was asked to lie on my side, curled up in the fetal position with my knees together and my shoulders straight. The doctor felt my spine to identify two of my lumbar vertebrae. I felt a cold sensation as the skin on my back was cleaned with antiseptic and then numbed with a local anesthetic. A needle was then passed between the bones in my back and through a

membrane to access the spinal fluid. The doctor had explained that it might feel uncomfortable but that it shouldn't be painful because there are no nerve endings in these layers; I was aware only of the pushing sensation of the needle in my back.

A nurse reassured me as the fluid dripped out of the needle into a collecting tube, which was sent off immediately for testing in the laboratory. Apparently, the nerves of the spinal cord finish two bones above the site of the puncture, so there is no

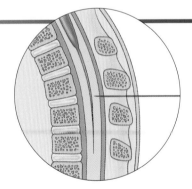

risk of damage or paralysis. Once the needle was removed, I sat up; it had all taken only a couple of minutes. I had a bit of a headache afterwards, which the doctor said was because of the lower pressure of the cerebrospinal fluid. I went home and rested and felt fine the next day.

Using X-rays and contrast media

Clear images of the bones of the skull and spine are easily captured by plain X-rays. To "see" the blood vessels lying underneath them, however, doctors combine X-rays with special radiopaque substances that are injected into the vessels to highlight them.

X-RAYS

Like radio waves and light waves, X-rays are a type of invisible electromagnetic short-wave radiation. X-ray images are shadow pictures that show the contrast between tissues of different density. Whether a part of the body shows up as white or gray depends on whether the X-rays can pass through it.

What are they used for?

X-ray images of the skull or spine can show any bone fractures or secondary deposits from cancer in bones adjacent to the brain and spinal cord. They are also useful for highlighting areas of dense tissue, such as tumors.

How do they work?

Produced using a device called an X-ray tube, X-rays are emitted as a single beam that is focused on the skull or an area of the spine positioned above a special cassette within an X-ray bed. The X-ray cassette contains either radiographic film or a substance that allows digital capture of the image, which can then be called up on a computer screen. X-rays are released from the tube for a fraction of a second and pass through the body into the cassette. Areas that absorb X-rays, such as the dense bone of the skull and spine, appear white, whereas less dense areas, such as brain tissue, absorb fewer rays and appear in varying shades of gray; air-filled structures, such as the nostrils, appear black because the X-rays pass straight through. The resulting X-ray image is the familiar "negative," which is examined by a radiologist on a light box.

Are there any adverse effects?

Having an X-ray carries no immediate risk and is a painless procedure. The radiation involved in taking an X-ray, though, may damage living cells and can lead to cancer. The effect of radiation is cumulative: The risk increases with repeated X-rays. For this reason, doctors and technicians monitor a person's exposure and always use the minimum possible for the best diagnostic result.

Particular parts of the body, such as the lens of the eye, the sperm cells in the testes, and the egg cells in the

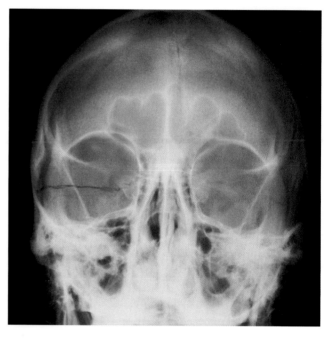

A fractured skull
The dense bone of the skull obscures the soft tissue of the brain inside. A fracture in the bone can be clearly seen here as a dark horizontal line on the left-hand side.

ovaries, are screened with lead aprons to shield them from X-rays. A woman is always asked if she is pregnant before having an X-ray because radiation during the first three months of pregnancy can result in fetal abnormalities.

CONTRAST X-RAYS

Some substances absorb X-rays much better than others. Medical experts have developed a way of exploiting this fact to create a more sophisticated diagnostic tool than the simple X-ray. Using substances called contrast media, which readily absorb X-rays, doctors can produce X-rays that highlight blood vessels or the cerebrospinal fluid surrounding the brain and spinal cord. The technique has different names, depending on what is under investigation:
- Angiography looks at blood vessels.
- Arteriography highlights arteries.
- Phlebography or venography visualises veins.

- Myelography shows the spinal cord and nerves arising from it.

What are they used for?

Imaging blood vessels of the brain—cerebral angiography—can help to diagnose a stroke (cerebrovascular disease) or a tumor. Arteriography is used mainly to investigate a "blow-out" of an artery—an aneurysm—or other causes of bleeding within the head.

How do they work?

For intra-arterial angiography of the brain, a neuroradiologist first injects a local anesthetic into the groin area. A fine plastic tube is then inserted into the femoral artery in the groin and pushed gently up through the arteries to the upper part of the aorta (the main artery leaving the heart) and on to the arteries supplying the tissues of the head and neck, including the brain. An iodine-containing contrast liquid is injected into the artery and a series of X-rays is taken, tracing the passage of the liquid through the vessels. The contrast medium absorbs X-rays strongly and highlights any abnormalities in the vessels. In myelography, the doctor injects contrast medium into the cerebrospinal fluid in a similar way to taking a lumbar puncture—between two vertebrae.

Are there any adverse effects?

Angiography carries a small risk of stroke because it involves placing a catheter in a main artery—its use is therefore restricted. An alternative is intravenous angiography, which injects a much larger volume of contrast medium into a vein. When the contrast eventually reaches the arteries in the neck and brain, a series of X-rays is taken. The procedure is safer than intra-arterial angiography, but the image quality is inferior.

Some people have adverse reactions to the contrast medium, and may feel nauseous or a flushing sensation. In addition, some conditions, such as hay fever, asthma, and diabetes, can be exacerbated by the procedure.

Looking under the skin

a The spidery network of blood vessels of this healthy brain are clearly highlighted on this cerebral angiogram.

b This contrast X-ray shows, from behind, a "ballooning out" of a blood vessel in the brain. Known as a berry aneurysm, this condition often requires surgery.

c This myelogram shows the spinal cord below the level of injection into the cerebrospinal fluid.

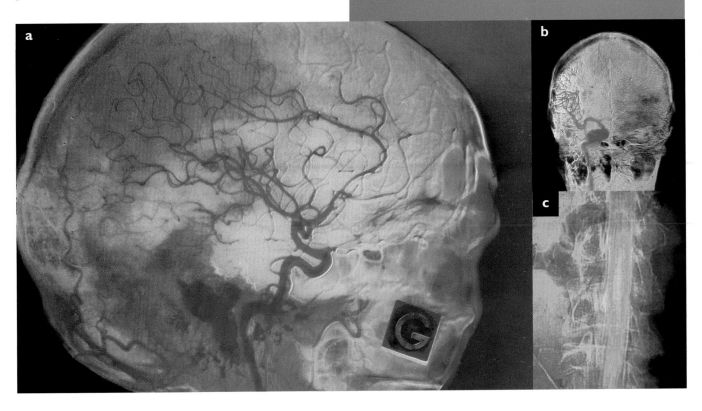

Brain scans—looking inside the skull

Doctors can now see inside our heads and produce detailed computerized pictures of the brain to show exactly what is going on underneath the bony skull. Sophisticated scanning techniques have already transformed the diagnosis of brain disorders, and the technology continues to improve.

COMPUTED TOMOGRAPHY (CT) SCANNING

Tomography, derived from the Greek *tomos*, means to draw by cutting, and is applied to many techniques in which a picture of a cross section or "slice" of the body is produced. CT scanning revolutionized brain investigation when it was introduced in the early 1970s; it was later applied to looking at the spine, but its main role remains in brain scanning. Just to show you how far the advance of computer technology has brought this imaging technique, in 1972 it took seven minutes to produce a single picture of a "slice" 1 centimeter thick, but now the latest CT scanner hardware and computer programs have developed to the extent that a whole head can be examined in just 90 seconds.

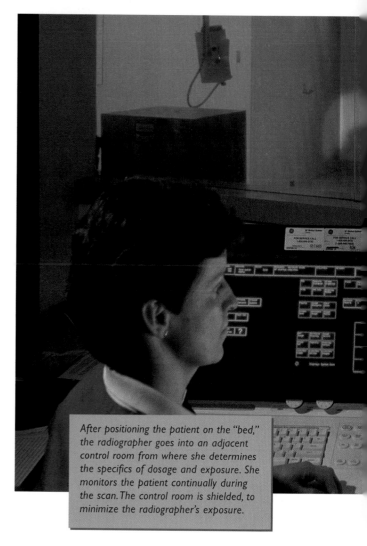

After positioning the patient on the "bed," the radiographer goes into an adjacent control room from where she determines the specifics of dosage and exposure. She monitors the patient continually during the scan. The control room is shielded, to minimize the radiographer's exposure.

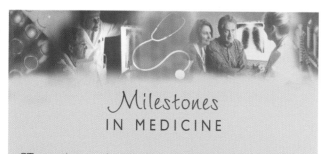

Milestones
IN MEDICINE

CT scanning was invented by a British physicist, Sir Godfrey Hounsfield, who won a Nobel prize for medicine for his revolutionary diagnostic technique. Because he was working for EMI (in London) at the time, the first model was known as the EMI scanner. Another name for CT is CAT, from its original technical name computed axial tomography. The detail CT scanning provided in its visualization of the brain was unprecedented, enabling doctors to make diagnoses more easily than ever before. CT scanning is now widely available and is the frontline diagnostic tool for investigations into brain disorders.

What is it used for?

Doctors use CT scanning when they suspect damage or change to structures inside the skull—as the result of head injury, hemorrhage, stroke or tumor. CT slices can show, for example, the minor differences in absorption of X-rays by areas affected by a stroke because of an increase in the proportion of water in that area.

How does it work?

An X-ray source on one side of the scanner sends a narrow beam of X-rays through the brain. These rays are picked up on the other side of the head by a very sensitive detector, which registers fine variations in tissue density and assigns each tissue type a shade of gray. By rotating the X-ray tube and the detectors around the head, the computer forms a cross-sectional "map" of the head using data on tissue absorption from different angles.

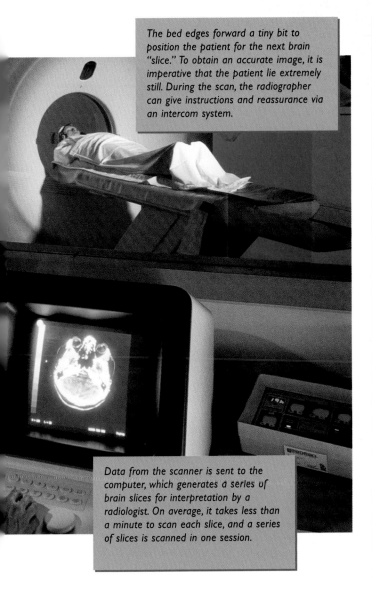

The bed edges forward a tiny bit to position the patient for the next brain "slice." To obtain an accurate image, it is imperative that the patient lie extremely still. During the scan, the radiographer can give instructions and reassurance via an intercom system.

Data from the scanner is sent to the computer, which generates a series of brain slices for interpretation by a radiologist. On average, it takes less than a minute to scan each slice, and a series of slices is scanned in one session.

Mapping the brain's infrastructure

a Using information from a series of brain slices, a computer can display different views, such as this vertical scan of a healthy brain and skull. Colors have been assigned to distinguish different brain structures from one another.

b This colored cross-sectional, or horizontal, brain slice shows an area of reduced blood flow, highlighted in red on the left. Regions of the brain with a normal blood supply are shown in green, and fluid-filled spaces within the brain are colored blue.

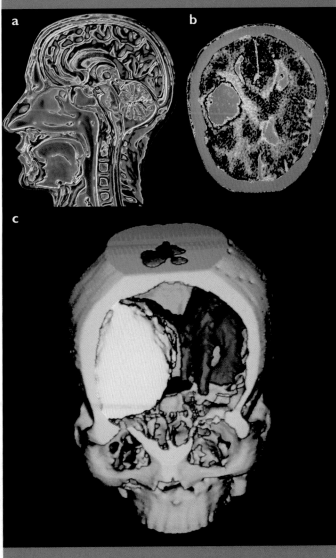

c Before operating, surgeons combine CT scans to build a 3-D model to find out exactly where a tumor lies (shown as yellow) relative to other parts of the brain.

Contrast media can be combined with CT to highlight blood vessels in the head or areas where the blood–brain barrier (see page 19) has broken down. The liquid contrast medium is injected into a vein in the arm while the person lies within the scanner.

Are there any adverse effects?

Radiation exposure during CT scans is comparatively low, but because a series of scans is usually taken, a person is exposed to more radiation in total than in a simple X-ray. To minimize exposure, CT scanners use very short bursts of radiation in a discrete beam. All X-rays are, however, a form of ionizing radiation, and repeated exposure can potentially lead to cancer. Before beginning contrast CT scanning, the technician will routinely ask about any conflicting conditions such as asthma, and about medication, to avoid any adverse effects.

MAGNETIC RESONANCE IMAGING (MRI)

This technique was introduced in the 1980s; one of its major advantages is that it does not use radiation known to be harmful to the body. It produces detailed cross-sectional images of the brain using a powerful magnetic field in conjunction with radio waves.

What is it used for?

An MRI scan produces a much more detailed image of the brain than CT scans, and clearly distinguishes between the brain's gray and white matter. MRI may be used to diagnose conditions such as multiple sclerosis, brain tumors, hemorrhage, and spinal cord damage.

MRI can also be adapted to measure blood flow and highlight vessels in the neck and head. Known as magnetic resonance angiography (MRA), this type of MRI is not as reliable as intra-arterial angiography (see page 105) because the images lack fine detail. Techniques are being refined, however, and, importantly, MRA carries no risks.

How does it work?

The heart of the imager is a large magnet, usually of "superconducting" type, with a strength between 10,000 and 30,000 times that of the earth's magnetic field. MRI exploits the fact that the majority of tissues in the body contain a certain amount of water; the hydrogen atoms within the water are the key to how it works. When placed in the strong magnetic field, the hydrogen atoms within the body line up—as though pointing to an imaginary North. These atoms are then "excited" by a short burst of radio waves, which makes them "wobble." As they recover and line up once more under the influence of the magnetic field, the nuclei of these atoms emit what is known as a "nuclear magnetic resonance signal." The imager detects these different signals and from the changes in the atoms' behavior can construct a map of the brain or spinal cord.

The examination consists of a number of "sequences," which give pictures or "slices" of the head in different

HAVING AN MRI BRAIN SCAN

When I arrived in the radiography department I was rather nervous; then I saw the MRI machine and I became even more worried.

I was sure that I would get claustrophobic with my head inside the scanner. The technician tried to make me feel more at ease, however, by explaining what was going to happen.

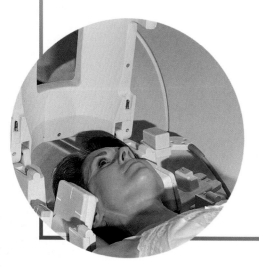

Before I entered the MRI room I had to take off all my jewelery, and I was asked if I had any removable dental braces or any metal within my body from previous operations or accidents—happily I don't. I left my handbag with the technician—she explained that all my credit cards and other items with magnetic strips would be affected by the magnetic field if I took them in with me. I was given some ear plugs as the scanner is noisy when it is in operation.

The technician positioned me on the bed and placed the coil around my head and then went into an adjoining room where she could monitor me through a window during the scan. She gave me a small alarm device to hold so that I could attract her attention if I felt uncomfortable, but I found I didn't

need it; she talked to me via the intercom throughout the examination, letting me know what she was doing, which was reassuring.

There were several sequences, each one recording a different "slice" of my brain—the technician told me each time a new sequence started, and how long it would take. Some sequences took longer than others and the machine made more noise—on average, a sequence lasted five minutes. During each scan, I had to keep my head as still as possible. I must have been fidgeting at one point, because the technician asked me to stop tapping my foot—apparently even movement this far away from the head can affect the scan. The whole examination took about half an hour.

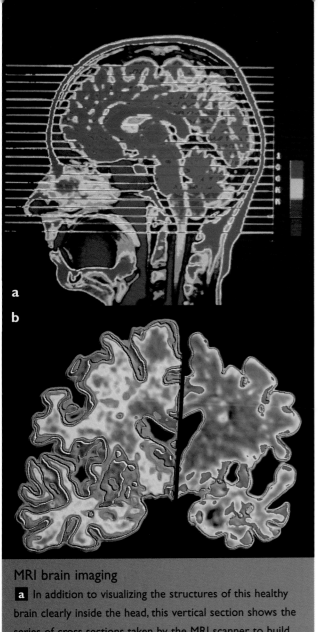

MRI brain imaging

a In addition to visualizing the structures of this healthy brain clearly inside the head, this vertical section shows the series of cross sections taken by the MRI scanner to build up the picture.

b By comparing it against a normal brain (*left*), it is possible to see how much the brain diminishes in the progressive degeneration of Alzheimer's disease (*right*).

AT THE LEADING EDGE

Functional MRI

When you use your brain to move a limb, for example, or to focus your eyes on something, the blood flow increases to the particular part of the brain concerned with that activity. This can be detected using MRI, as increased oxygen levels around the activated tissue change the magnetic resonance signal. The manner in which the normal movement of water molecules in the brain (called diffusion) is influenced by disease can be investigated by diffusion-weighted MRI. This new technique promises to be of value in detecting stroke, possibly at a very early stage when it may be feasible to give treatment to limit damage to the brain. Perfusion imaging—another type of MRI—can be used to examine what happens as a contrast medium, injected into an arm vein, passes through the brain. Experts hope that these MRI developments will be of great benefit for diagnosing stroke and brain tumors.

directions, or are adjusted in order to look at different characteristics of the tissues.

The drawback to MRI scanning is that the conditions required to construct maps of "slices" of the body analogous to those produced by a CT scanner are extremely demanding. An MRI scanner is therefore much larger, more complex, and considerably more expensive than a CT scanner. From the patient's point of view, the examination is also much longer in duration—it may take two or three minutes for each slice to be produced.

Like CT, MRI may involve an injection of contrast medium into a vein. Here the substance usually contains a magnetically influenced element called gadolinium rather than iodine as used with CT.

Are there any adverse effects?

Because the magnetic field of the imager is incredibly strong, it can affect heart pacemakers (which contain small switches), metallic clips used to seal off a blood vessel within the head, and hearing implants in the inner ear. A metal fragment lodged in the body as the result of an accident may also move in the magnetic field and cause damage to tissues as it moves around. Anyone for whom a doctor has requested an MRI will therefore be asked questions to ensure that it is safe to proceed.

Some people find lying with their head at the center of the tunnel produces feelings of claustrophobia, but most individuals are able to tolerate a scanning session. Those who are particularly nervous are sometimes given a mild sedative. Occasionally, if it is necessary to carry out an MRI on young children, or on adults who are mentally disturbed or whose illness means they cannot keep still, a general anesthetic is given. Side effects from the contrast medium gadolinium are very rare.

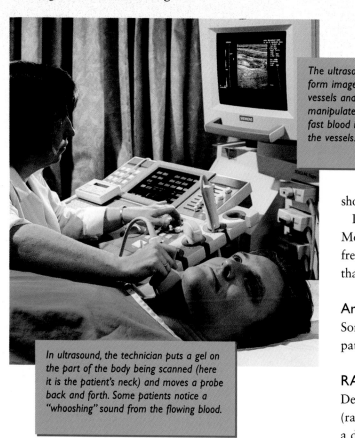

The ultrasound machine can form images of the blood vessels and can also be manipulated to measure how fast blood is flowing through the vessels.

In ultrasound, the technician puts a gel on the part of the body being scanned (here it is the patient's neck) and moves a probe back and forth. Some patients notice a "whooshing" sound from the flowing blood.

ULTRASOUND SCANNING

Also known as sonography, ultrasound scanning does not employ dangerous radiation. Indeed, the safety of the technique is such that most pregnant women have an ultrasound scan of the womb to check the baby's size and to look for abnormalities, such as spina bifida.

What is it used for?

Sound waves pass very poorly through bone, but because babies have gaps in their skull bones—acoustic windows—ultrasound scanning can be used to detect damage to the brain. In adults, a type of sonography called Doppler ultrasound can be used to investigate blood flow to the brain and to detect obstructions or narrowing in any vital blood vessels. Many strokes occur in people who have narrowing and irregularity of the lining of arteries in the neck, caused by hardening of the arteries. The risk of further strokes can be reduced by identifying the damaged segment of a blood vessel and widening or replacing it.

How does it work?

The physical basis of sonography is the same as that of radar, in which sound waves bounce off objects. To examine the carotid artery, a probe emitting sound waves is pressed against the neck. The sound waves reflect off the body's tis-

sues as "echoes," which are received by the same probe. Different tissues reflect the sound waves to different degrees. Because the probe also determines how long the waves take to return to it, the position of these tissues in space can be determined. A built-in computer builds a picture showing the anatomical relationship of the various structures.

Doppler sonography makes use of the "Doppler effect": Moving particles, such as the cells in the blood, change the frequency of the sound waves they reflect in the same way that the siren of a police car drops in pitch as it passes.

Are there any adverse effects?

Sonography has no known risks. It is used to select patients for more detailed investigation.

RADIONUCLIDE SCANNING

Detection of radioactive chemical compounds (radionuclides) introduced into the body has been used as a diagnostic method for about 40 years; it is used to examine function rather than structure. Its use in diagnosis of certain conditions has largely been supplanted by CT scanning and MRI. More sophisticated techniques, such as single-photon emission computed tomography (SPECT) and positron emission tomography (PET) can be used to investigate brain function, but are used more often as research tools than in everyday diagnosis.

What is it used for?

Radionuclide scanning is used mainly for detecting patterns of brain dysfunction or tumors within the brain. It is sometimes used to identify the source of an epileptic seizure, or in the diagnosis of rare causes of dementia

How does it work?

A radionuclide-containing substance is injected into a vein or sometimes inhaled as a gas. These chemicals travel to the brain and emit a type of radiation known as gamma rays, which can be detected using a radiation-sensitive device. A tumor, for example, can be located by its unusual uptake of the gamma-labeled radionuclide.

Are there any adverse effects?

Radionuclides emit only small amounts of radiation, so the technique is very safe. But as with any procedure involving radiation, exposure is closely monitored.

Measuring the brain's electricity

The brain works via electricity, which can be measured by electroencephalography—EEG. It was once the standard investigation for neurological disease, and, although it is now used less, it remains an essential tool in finding out how the brain is functioning.

What is an EEG used for?

Every neuron in the body communicates via electrical and chemical signals. Recording the brain waves made by the electrical signals in the brain can help in the diagnosis of neurological conditions such as epilepsy, certain types of encephalitis, dementia, and brain tumors.

Wave patterns that are different from normal can be characteristic of particular neurological diseases.

- Spikes or sharp waves may be seen in people with epilepsy between seizures. During an epileptic seizure the EEG may be abnormal over the whole brain (generalized epilepsy) or in one anatomically restricted area (focal epilepsy).
- Brain waves disappear altogether if there has been massive brain damage, such as prolonged oxygen starvation after a heart attack or partial drowning. This phenomenon may also be seen in someone who has taken barbiturate drugs or is suffering from hypothermia.
- Slow waves, characteristically over the temporal lobes, may be associated with viral encephalitis.

If you could harness the electricity generated by the neurons in your brain, you could light up a 20-watt lightbulb.

- An EEG of someone with Creutzfeldt–Jacob Disease has bursts of high-amplitude sharp waves; in contrast, an EEG of someone with Alzheimer's would have few variations.

How does it work?

An EEG machine records the spontaneous electrical activity (as voltages over time) generated by nerve cells in the cerebral cortex. The EEG trace is a series of waves; different rhythms are characteristic of different parts of the brain. The cortex is also influenced by nerve connections from other brain structures, such as the thalamus, and their combined activities generate the rhythms of the brainwaves.

Sometimes, a person may have EEG monitoring combined with video recording for several days to determine whether or not the diagnosis is epilepsy.

Are there any adverse effects?

An EEG is a simple and painless procedure; no shaving of the head is necessary and there are no side effects.

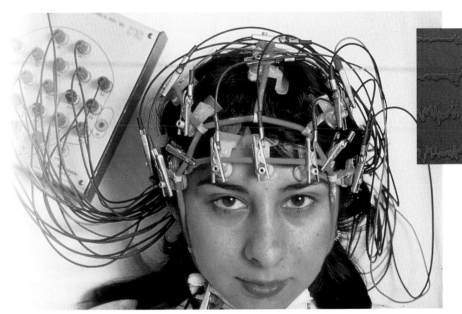

Having an EEG
An EEG is recorded, usually while the subject sits in a chair with closed eyes, using electrodes attached to the head with sticky jelly that is able to conduct electricity. Multiple electrodes measure several areas of the brain at the same time to create a map of global brain activity.

Taking a tissue sample—biopsy

A biopsy involves removing a sample of tissue or cells from the body, which is then sent off for microscopic examination in the laboratory. Because of the delicacy of neurological structures, biopsy is performed only when absolutely necessary.

TEMPORAL ARTERY

Temporal arteritis is an inflammatory disorder that can affect the arteries to the brain and the eye, leading to stroke and blindness, respectively. Once identified, the condition is easily treatable with steroid drugs. Although the symptoms of scalp tenderness and headache are characteristic, the definitive test is to remove a segment of the temporal artery to look for inflammation. This artery arises from the external carotid artery and passes up to the scalp just in front of the ear over the temple. This area of scalp receives blood from other vessels, so this artery segment can be removed without any harm. A surgeon performs the biopsy under local anesthetic.

BRAIN TISSUE

In general, the brain is biopsied only from sites that can be reached with minimal damage to normal brain tissue and only in the following circumstances.

- Brain tumor A biopsy can establish whether the tumour is benign or malignant and whether it originates directly from brain tissue or from elsewhere in the body.
- Infective abnormality where the organism is in question Tuberculosis, for example, may cause areas of inflammation in the brain; such unusual infections can sometimes only be diagnosed by biopsy.

These biopsies are conducted under general anaesthetic.

PERIPHERAL NERVE

Occasionally, it is impossible for a doctor to uncover the cause of peripheral nerve disease despite nerve electrical studies and detailed blood tests. In this situation, a nerve biopsy may be necessary to exclude inflammatory disease of the nerve blood vessels, which may require drugs to suppress the body's immune system. The usual nerve biopsied is one found on the outside of the foot—the sural nerve. Once removed, there is a small patch of numbness and the area may be painful for a while afterwards.

MUSCLE TISSUE

Messages from the brain are relayed to the muscles via nerves, so doctors want to rule out an infection or inflammation affecting muscle tissue, which could be

Comparing nerve tissue

a *This sample contains healthy cells taken from the outer layer of the brain—the cerebral cortex.*
b *In sharp contrast, these adenocarcinoma cells taken from a brain biopsy confirm the presence of a tumor.*

Comparing muscle tissue

c *This microscopic photograph shows normal muscle fibers.*
d *An inflammatory disease, such as polymyositis, destroys the orderly arrangement of these fibers; this specimen clearly highlights a problem.*

confused with a neurological problem. Muscle biopsy—often from the quadriceps in the thigh—must be taken carefully from a site affected by the disease but not in such an advanced stage that the muscle has been totally destroyed. Analysis determines the presence of an infection, such as toxoplasmosis, or an inflammation, such as polymyositis. Tissue specimens can be stained for the dystrophin protein, which is absent in muscular dystrophy.

Because of increasing accuracy and adaptability of imaging techniques such as MRI, together with improvements in laboratory tests and genetic analysis, the demand for biopsy is likely to continue to diminish.

CURRENT TREATMENTS

Powerful drugs, accurate and effective surgery, and efficient rehabilitation programs all contribute to the many successes in neurological medicine. Recent advances in medication have meant that people with conditions such as Parkinson's disease, epilepsy, and some psychological disorders can live normal lives. Surgical techniques, too, are developing to such an extent that brain tumors can now be removed with pinpoint accuracy. Where drugs and surgery are not appropriate, people who have suffered disabling brain damage can now often regain their independence with a tailormade rehabilitation program.

Drugs for the nervous system

Treatment for central nervous system disorders has advanced rapidly in recent years as our understanding of the human brain has improved, and there are now many effective drug therapies available.

PAIN-RELIEVING DRUGS

Analgesic drugs, better known as painkillers, alleviate pain, but don't usually treat the underlying cause of the pain. Most analgesics are taken in tablet form, but sometimes they are given as injections or suppositories.

How do they work?

Chemicals called prostaglandins are released by cells in the damaged area, triggering nearby nerve endings to send messages to pain receptors in the brain. Prostaglandins can also cause inflammation at the injured site. Analgesics either prevent the production of prostaglandins or they

Tips for drug safety

The majority of people taking drugs suffer no side effects at all. Of those that do, the response to the same drug varies immensely and can range from a slight feeling of nausea to a severe allergic reaction. Whatever the reaction, the advice to the patient is the same: If new symptoms appear that seem to be related to taking drugs, go straight back to the doctor.

Always read the information on the package BEFORE you begin taking the medication, particularly as it may suggest taking drugs with food or advise what to do if a dose is missed. Never exceed or reduce the dose recommended without seeking medical advice.

Some medications can interact with other drugs, including over-the-counter ones, or with alcohol to produce unpleasant side effects. Check the package or ask the doctor or pharmacist.

Children, pregnant women, and the elderly may all need reduced doses of many drugs, and some drugs should be avoided altogether. If in doubt, check with the doctor or pharmacist.

The same drug may be available under different names, depending on the manufacturer. In most cases, this book uses the approved (generic) name for a drug, not the trade name.

block the pain receptors in the brain. They are categorized into non-opioid and opioid drugs.

- **Non-opioid drugs** Nonsteroidal antiinflammatory drugs (NSAIDs), which include aspirin and ibuprofen, block prostaglandin production at the pain site. Acetaminophen, one of the most commonly used analgesics, works in the same way as opioid drugs by reducing the perception of pain in the brain.
- **Opioid drugs** These block the passage of pain signals inside the brain. Opioids, for example morphine and codeine, are stronger drugs and are often prescribed for people with sudden, severe pain, for example during a heart attack or following surgery or trauma. They are also prescribed for long-term worsening pain when weaker painkillers are no longer effective.

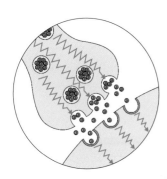

Blocking the pain
Electrical impulses travel along nerve pathways from the site of the pain. Where one nerve cell meets the next, chemicals (red circles) relay the pain message to receptors in the brain (above). Many analgesics (brown triangles, below) act by blocking pain receptors so that the signals cannot continue their journey.

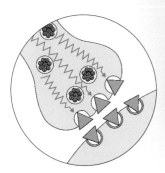

What are the adverse effects?

In normal circumstances, acetaminophen is very safe at the recommended dosage. Exceeding this dose, however, can cause irreversible liver damage; a person who already has a liver problem should avoid taking acetaminophen. NSAIDs can sometimes cause indigestion, ulcers or bleeding in the gut. Taking the drugs with food or using stomach-protecting medication should reduce this risk. Aspirin should never be given to children under 12 because of the risk of the drug leading to a rare disorder called Reye's syndrome, which affects the liver and brain.

Constipation is common in people taking opioid drugs, as is nausea and dizziness. Stronger opioids may cause breathing difficulties, drowsiness, and confusion. If used for a long time, the dose may stop being effective and dependence can develop.

DRUGS FOR NAUSEA AND VOMITING

Within the brain is an area known as the vomiting center, which when stimulated gives rise to the symptoms of nausea and vomiting. Doctors sometimes prescribe anti-nauseant tablets to counteract these symptoms. If the symptoms are severe, and a person is unable to hold the tablets down, the drugs can also be given in injection form or as suppositories, which are inserted into the rectum.

How do they work?

The vomiting center receives messages from, and is stimulated by, various areas of the body, such as the chemoreceptor trigger zone in the brain (which is sensitive to chemicals in the bloodstream), the inner ear, and the stomach. Drugs act on one or more of these areas to prevent messages from reaching the vomiting center.

- **Dopamine receptor antagonists** These drugs block chemoreceptors in the brain, which detect the nerve impulses that indicate nausea. Examples include metoclopramide, domperidone, and prochlorperazine.
- **Hyoscine hydrobromide** A useful drug for travel sickness, this is most effective when taken before the start of a journey. It should not, however, be taken by someone who intends to drive. The drug can be applied as a tiny patch behind the ear to enable continuous release of the medication.

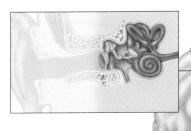

The brain's vomiting center
Abrupt changes in balance or orientation are relayed to the vomiting center from the inner ear, hence the feeling of nausea related to travel or motion.

How do they work?

Migraine drugs reverse the vasodilation in the brain by narrowing the arteries, a process known as vasoconstriction. Different drugs have different actions, but they all work toward producing the same effect. Drugs used solely in the treatment (not prevention) of migraine attacks include:

• **Ergotamine tartrate** A powerful vasoconstrictor of blood vessels in the outer area of the brain; it works best when taken during the early stages of an attack.

• **Serotonin agonists (triptans)** These are the newest agents developed for the treatment of migraine. Experts believe that when levels of the neurotransmitter serotonin fall below normal, they trigger vasodilation in the arteries and thus a migraine attack. These drugs boost serotonin levels and therefore reverse the vasodilation.

Medicines to prevent attacks from occurring include:

• **Beta-blockers** These are normally used to lower blood pressure, but they have also been shown to help in the prevention of migraine.

• **Antihistamines** These drugs help to control nausea due to balance disturbance. They work by acting on sites in the inner ear, which relay messages to the brain.

• **Serotonin receptor antagonists** These are particularly useful in preventing and treating the nausea and vomiting that result from chemotherapy and radiotherapy treatment. They work by blocking the brain's serotonin receptors. Ondansetron is one example.

What are the adverse effects?

These drugs tend to produce side effects only with prolonged use, although most of them cause drowsiness. People taking serotonin receptor antagonists commonly report headaches. Less frequently, constipation or diarrhea, fatigue, and dizziness may develop. Hyoscine may cause dry mouth, blurred vision, and dizziness.

DRUGS FOR MIGRAINE

The pain of migraine is caused by a widening (vasodilation) of blood vessels in the brain. The reason for this is unclear, but experts believe that certain chemical imbalances may play a part. If a migraine does not respond to simple analgesic drugs, such as acetaminophen or nonsteroidal antiinflammatories, a specific migraine drug can be used either to treat attacks or to prevent future ones.

Migraine drugs come in capsule, tablet, suppository (which are inserted into the rectum), injection, "wafer" (which dissolves in the mouth), or nasal spray forms.

A migraine strikes
The pain of a migraine can be debilitating, and even strong painkillers are often ineffective. Migraine drugs act to narrow the dilated blood vessels in the brain that are thought to cause the symptoms.

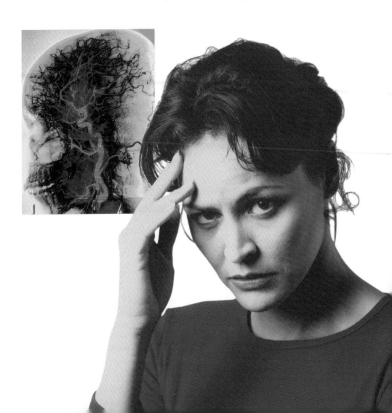

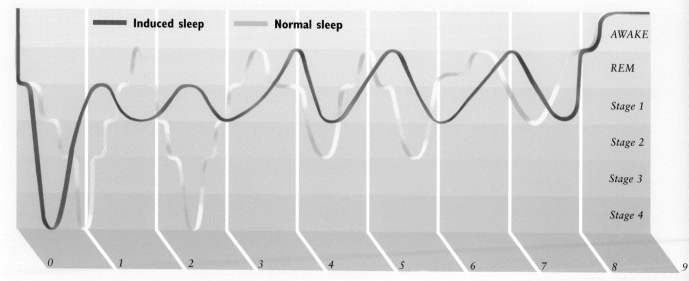

Induced sleep   **Normal sleep**

AWAKE

REM

Stage 1

Stage 2

Stage 3

Stage 4

0   1   2   3   4   5   6   7   8   9

Hours of sleep

- **Tricyclic antidepressants** These drugs affect levels of serotonin in the brain and are sometimes tried in low doses to treat migraine.

What are the adverse effects?
Many of the drugs used to treat migraine can cause drowsiness, nausea, or changes in bowel habit. In addition, serotonin agonists may cause dizziness and flushing. If a feeling of tightness in the throat or chest develops, the doctor will probably stop the drug. Beta-blockers can cause coldness of the extremities and sleep disturbances, including nightmares. Blurred vision is sometimes experienced with tricyclic antidepressants.

SLEEPING DRUGS
Insomnia is the inability to sleep or to stay asleep. Sleeping drugs—hypnotics—can often help, but it is important that the reason for insomnia is established before any medication is prescribed. Hypnotic drugs are available as tablets, capsules, and in liquid form.

How do they work?
All hypnotic drugs attach themselves to receptors found on nerves in the brain. This increases the effects of a brain chemical called GABA, which inhibits transmission of electrical signals along the nerves within the brain. As a result, overall brain activity slows down, promoting sleep. The following drugs are used to achieve this effect.
- **Benzodiazepines** These are widely prescribed for insomnia, and they also relieve anxiety.

Induced sleep patterns
Sleep induced by drugs (hypnotics) has a distinctive pattern and lacks much of the deep sleep element of a normal night's rest. In addition, REM sleep is suppressed. A person taking hypnotics commonly feels unrefreshed and slightly groggy on waking.

- **Chloral hydrate** This is particularly useful for the elderly, because it is free from any "hangover effect."
- **Zolpidem** This is a recently developed hypnotic that works in the same way as benzodiazepines, but has little or no "hangover effect."
- **Antihistamines** Although these are not specifically hypnotic drugs, they are sometimes used for insomnia, particularly in children, because drowsiness is a side effect. Many of these can be bought over the counter, but advice from the pharmacist is recommended.

What are the adverse effects?
If hypnotics are taken long term, the dose may become ineffective, or dependence on the drug may develop, so doctors advise using them for only short periods of time (usually one to four weeks). If the drugs are withdrawn suddenly after long-term use, insomnia may return.

With many sleeping drugs—particularly benzodiazepines—drowsiness, lethargy, and a "hangover" effect may occur the next day, so it is unwise to drive or use machinery. People taking zolpidem may experience nausea or a nasty taste in the mouth.

DRUGS FOR ANXIETY

Anxiety is a feeling of tension and apprehension that is either present all the time or occurs as a sudden panic attack. The distressing symptoms of anxiety, such as palpitations, sweating, and shakiness, can be treated with drugs known as anxiolytics. These drugs will not cure the anxiety, so they should always be used together with other supportive therapies such as psychotherapy. Anxiolytics are most commonly prescribed as tablets or capsules but are also available as injections and oral solutions.

How do they work?

Chemical substances in the brain called neurotransmitters help messages pass from nerve to nerve. When a person is anxious, certain neurotransmitters become imbalanced and the brain becomes abnormally active. Drugs can be used to block or slow down this increased activity and thereby relieve the physical nature of the anxiety.

- **Benzodiazepines** These increase the actions of a particular neurotransmitter in the brain called GABA, high levels of which slow down the overactive brain. One example is diazepam, better known as Valium.
- **Buspirone** This scales down activity in the brain by decreasing the effects of the neurotransmitter serotonin. It has fewer side effects than the benzodiazepines, although it takes longer to work.
- **Beta-blockers** These drugs interfere with neuro-transmitters in the brain, heart, and muscles to reduce the physical symptoms of anxiety such as palpitations and tremor. The most commonly used beta-blocker is propranolol.

What are the adverse effects?

The main drawback of the benzodiazepines is that they can cause drowsiness, and in some people, dizziness and confusion, so they should only be used in the short term. Also, if these drugs are used for a long time, the dose can become ineffective and dependence may develop. Buspirone does not carry the risk of dependence, but occasionally people experience dizziness, headaches, or stomach upsets. Beta-blockers are generally well tolerated but can cause coldness of the fingers and toes, and sleep disturbances.

DRUGS FOR DEPRESSION

Depression is thought to be caused by low levels of the chemical substances in the brain—neurotransmitters—that are involved in message transmission. Some of these chemicals, particularly serotonin and norepinephrine, increase activity in the brain and so improve mood. Antidepressants are usually given as tablets or capsules, although injection and oral mixtures are also available.

How do they work?

Antidepressant drugs either behave like a neurotrans-mitter or boost its level. The response takes several weeks, so a lift in mood may not be seen immediately.

- **Selective serotonin reuptake inhibitors (SSRIs)** This is a group of drugs that blocks the reabsorption of serotonin by nerves, leaving more to stimulate brain cells and improve mood. A well-known example is Prozac.
- **Tricyclic antidepressants (TCAs)** These interfere with the reabsorption of serotonin and norepinephrine, so that the levels of these neurotransmitters remain high and their stimulatory effect is prolonged.
- **Monoamine oxidase inhibitors (MAOIs)** These block the action of an enzyme, monoamine oxidase, which inactivates excess neurotransmitters, thereby boosting their levels. Certain foods and drugs can interfere with MAOIs, and the doctor should advise on what to avoid.

Chemical messengers in the brain
This greatly magnified image shows crystals of the neurotransmitter serotonin, which helps to pass messages from nerve to nerve. Experts believe that low levels of serotonin can lead to depression and anxiety.

What are the adverse effects?

At the start of treatment with SSRIs, people often feel nauseated and have diarrhea. TCAs can cause blurred vision, dry mouth, constipation, and difficulty passing urine. People taking MAOIs may experience these same side effects as well as weight gain, headaches, and drowsiness.

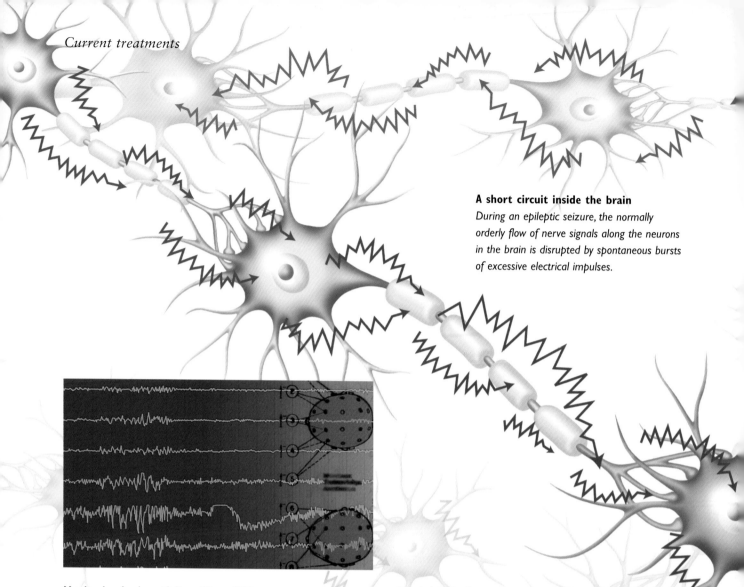

A short circuit inside the brain
During an epileptic seizure, the normally orderly flow of nerve signals along the neurons in the brain is disrupted by spontaneous bursts of excessive electrical impulses.

Monitoring brain activity with an EEG
This electroencephalogram (EEG) tracing shows the electrical activity in the brain of a person with epilepsy. An episode of frantic activity at the start of the tracing confirms a brief epileptic seizure, which is soon followed by a return to normal.

DRUGS FOR EPILEPSY

In epilepsy, abnormal electrical activity in the brain causes seizures. Anticonvulsant drugs are prescribed to prevent seizures from occurring or to reduce their frequency and severity. For these drugs to be effective, it is important that they are taken regularly and at the times suggested, even if a seizure has not occurred for a while. Doctors can prescribe the drugs as tablets, capsules, liquid, suppositories (into the rectum), or as an injection.

How do they work?

Anticonvulsant drugs prevent the spread of abnormal, excessive electrical impulses along the nerves to other areas of the brain. Some drugs increase the amounts of GABA (gamma-amino butyric acid), a neurotransmitter that inhibits the passage of nerve signals. Other drugs alter the nerves themselves, again preventing the passage of electrical activity.

No single drug will control all types of seizures, and anyone suffering from epilepsy will be individually assessed before treatment begins. Initially, only one drug will be prescribed, depending on the type and severity of the seizures. If the selected drug fails to control the seizures, as occurs in some cases, the doctor may need to prescribe an alternative. Occasionally, more than one drug is required. Measuring the level of some drugs in the blood enables careful adjustments in the dose to be made, especially if the drug does not seem to be working as expected.

The oldest and still the most widely used drugs are phenytoin, carbamazepine, and sodium valproate. They are highly effective and are used to control different types of seizures. If these drugs do not control the epilepsy, newer drugs, such as lamotrigine or gabapentin, may help.

In the rare event of a prolonged, life-threatening seizure (status epilepticus) diazepam, commonly known as Valium, will be given intravenously.

What are the adverse effects?

Most anticonvulsant drugs can cause drowsiness, dizziness, headache, nausea and vomiting, muscle twitches, and tremors, especially when a person first begins treatment. These side effects are usually temporary and improve or disappear as the treatment continues. However, it is important to inform the doctor of any unusual fever, sore throat, bleeding, or bruising, as some drugs occasionally affect the immune system.

DRUGS FOR PARKINSON'S DISEASE

In Parkinson's disease an imbalance develops between two vital chemicals, acetylcholine and dopamine, which are responsible for sending messages to the part of the brain that coordinates movement. Levels of dopamine fall so that acetylcholine predominates, producing the distressing symptoms of tremor and muscle stiffness. The drugs used to treat Parkinson's disease only relieve the symptoms and cannot slow the progression of the disease or cure it.

How do they work?

Drug treatment is taken orally or given as injections and restores chemical balance by increasing levels of dopamine or blocking the effects of acetylcholine.

- **Levodopa** Once inside the brain, levodopa (the most commonly used drug) is broken down into dopamine, boosting its levels.
- **Carbidopa and benserazide** One of these drugs is usually given in conjunction with levodopa to prevent this chemical from being broken down before it reaches its target site—the brain.
- **COMT and MAOB inhibitors** These are sometimes given together with levodopa because they prevent its breakdown in the brain and therefore prolong its action.
- **Dopamine agonists** This group of drugs acts in the brain to mimic and boost the effects of dopamine. Bromocriptine, cabergoline, and pergolide are all examples of dopamine agonists.
- **Anticholinergics** These reduce acetylcholine levels by blocking its receptors on the nerve cells. They are effective at reducing tremor and muscle stiffness if tolerated at a sufficient dose.

What are the adverse effects?

Levodopa often causes nausea and vomiting, so the doctor may well prescribe an anti-nauseant tablet to be taken in conjunction with the drug. If the dose of levodopa is too high, it may cause involuntary movements of the face and body. Long-term use can lead to intermittent "freezing" for a period of time before mobility returns; it can also result in hallucinations and confusion. Dopamine agonists have similar side effects to levodopa, but there is a greater tendency to develop mental disturbance. Anticholinergics can cause a dry mouth, constipation, blurred vision, and memory loss.

DRUGS FOR SCHIZOPHRENIA

The psychotic symptoms of schizophrenia—thought disorders, hallucinations, and delusions—are believed to be the result of unusually high amounts of neurotransmitter chemicals in the brain, which normally help to pass messages along the nerve pathways. Drugs to treat these symptoms are known as antipsychotic drugs.

How do they work?

The drugs prevent the neurotransmitters dopamine and serotonin from having an effect on the brain by blocking their receptor sites. There are two main groups of drugs: standard antipsychotic drugs that block the dopamine receptors, and atypical antipsychotic drugs, which block both serotonin and dopamine receptors.

If standard or atypical antipsychotic drugs prove ineffective or produce side effects, newer drugs such as clozapine may be prescribed.

Not until the 1950s did doctors discover effective drugs for mental illness. Until then, sufferers were often locked in institutions with no hope for the future.

What are the adverse effects?

People taking standard antipsychotic drugs may experience tremor, restlessness, abnormal face and body movements, and slowed movements. These symptoms are collectively known as extrapyramidal side effects (EPSE) and can be reversed by taking anticholinergic drugs, but these may in turn cause a dry mouth, blurred vision, and stomach upsets. Atypical antipsychotics are less likely to cause EPSE, but are associated with weight gain, drowsiness, and dizziness. Regular blood tests are essential during treatment with clozapine because it can cause serious abnormalities in the blood.

Drugs to prevent stroke

Although stroke affects the brain, the causes occur in the circulatory system. Anyone, therefore, who has high blood pressure or raised cholesterol levels, or who has had a heart attack in the past, may be prescribed drugs to reduce the risk of stroke.

DRUGS FOR HIGH BLOOD PRESSURE

Consistently raised blood pressure (hypertension) can be caused either by an underlying disease that causes narrowing of the blood vessels or by abnormal regulation of salt and water in the circulation. Without treatment with anti-hypertensive drugs, a person with high blood pressure runs the risk of developing further complications such as stroke, heart disease, or kidney problems. The drugs exist in tablet, capsule, and injection form.

How do they work?

High blood pressure drugs work in one of two ways— either they act on the heart and blood vessels, or they increase the removal of salt from the circulation. Many different antihypertensive drugs are available, and often more than one drug is taken at a time. Commonly used antihypertensive drugs include the following:

- **Thiazide diuretics** These act on the kidneys to increase the amount of water and salt that they remove from the blood, thereby reducing the circulating volume.

Control of blood pressure
Some drugs relax the muscles in the walls of the arteries, increasing the diameter and elasticity of the vessels. This reduces the resistance that the vessel exerts on the blood and blood pressure falls.

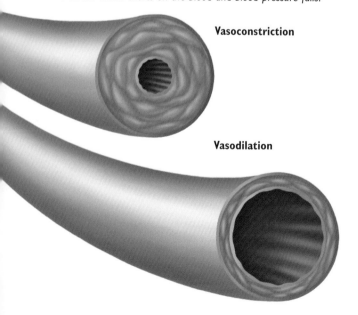

Vasoconstriction

Vasodilation

- **Calcium-channel blockers** These act directly on the muscles of the blood vessels to dilate them.
- **Beta-blockers** By acting directly on the heart, these reduce the force, and so pressure, at which blood is pumped around the body.
- **ACE inhibitors** These drugs dilate blood vessels by blocking the actions of angiotensin II, a naturally occurring chemical that makes blood vessels constrict. ACE is short for angiotensin converting enzyme.

What are the adverse effects?

Most antihypertensive drugs cause dizziness at the beginning of treatment as the blood pressure starts to drop. In addition, thiazide diuretics can lead to cramps because of a loss of body salts through the increased volume of urine. Taking calcium-channel blockers can result in swollen ankles, flushing, and headaches. Beta-blockers can cause a slow heart beat and cold fingers and toes. ACE inhibitors may produce a dry cough and headache.

DRUGS THAT AFFECT BLOOD CLOTTING

Blood clots usually form only in response to some type of injury, such as an accident, or surgery. Some people, however, have a high risk of forming a blood clot (thrombosis), which could block the blood supply to a vital organ, such as the brain or heart.

How do they work?

There are two ways to prevent damage caused by blood clots, thereby reducing the risk of stroke or heart disease—by preventing clots from forming (with anticoagulant or antiplatelet drugs) or by dissolving already existing clots (with thrombolytic drugs).

- **Anticoagulant drugs** These drugs prevent clot formation, stabilize existing clots, and prevent fragments of the clot from breaking off and traveling elsewhere in the body to block a blood vessel. These drugs come in two forms: those given intravenously (heparin) for an immediate effect and those given orally (coumadin), which take a few days to work and are used as a preventive treatment for people at risk of stroke.

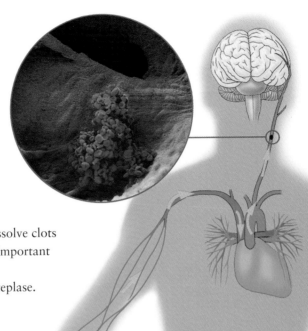

- **Antiplatelet drugs** These drugs reduce the stickiness of the tiny blood cells called platelets that help in blood clotting. Aspirin has an antiplatelet action and is commonly prescribed following a heart attack or stroke.
- **Thrombolytic drugs** These increase the amounts of an enzyme in the blood called plasmin that breaks down fibrin, one of the constituents of a blood clot. These drugs dissolve clots that have already formed and are blocking important vessels either to the brain or to the heart. Thrombolytics include streptokinase and alteplase.

What are the adverse effects?

The main risk of thrombolytic drugs is the increased likelihood of bleeding. Occasionally, nausea or an allergic reaction may develop.

Stabilizing a clot

An anticoagulant drug (indicated in green) can be injected into a vein in the arm to prevent a blood clot from growing bigger. If the clot, shown here in the main artery to the brain, were to enlarge or break off, it could cause a stroke.

Anticoagulant alert

If you are taking an anticoagulant drug, you have the potential to bleed more easily than other people. Consider wearing a Medic-Alert bracelet, in case you are in an accident or need surgery. Contact your doctor if you answer "yes" to any of these questions.

- *Are you bruising badly, even in places you didn't know you had bumped?*
- *Have you noticed blood in your urine or stools?*
- *Is your nose bleeding spontaneously?*
- *Are there small broken blood vessels on the whites of your eyes?*

LIPID-LOWERING DRUGS

Some lipids (fats), notably cholesterol and triglycerides, can build up in the blood and form fatty plaques in the arteries—atherosclerosis. If the plaques restrict the blood supply to the brain or the heart, a stroke or heart attack could occur. If lipid levels are not lowered significantly by a change in diet, then lipid-lowering drugs may be given to reduce levels and prevent further build-up of fats.

How do they work?

Lipid-lowering drugs act on the digestive system to reduce blood cholesterol and/or triglycerides.

- **Anion-exchange resins** These chemicals bind with cholesterol in the intestine and prevent its absorption. They include cholestyramine and colestipol.
- **Fibrates** Their action focuses on the liver, where they block production of several different lipids, including triglycerides and cholesterol. Gemfibrozil is one example.
- **Statins** These drugs block enzymes in the liver to prevent the manufacture of cholesterol. Examples of statins include simvastatin and pravastatin.

What are the adverse effects?

Anion-exchange resins are not absorbed into the bloodstream, but they may cause digestive problems such as constipation, nausea, and vomiting. They can also inhibit the absorption of other drugs. Rarely, fibrates and statins can cause muscle pain or weakness.

Electroconvulsive therapy (ECT)

ECT was first developed in the 1930s when doctors made a chance discovery that in some people who had both epilepsy and mental illness, an epileptic seizure would lead to an improvement in their mental health.

WHAT IS ECT?
ECT is now only carried out using a general anesthetic and drugs that relax the muscles. A small electric current is passed across the brain for about 2 to 3 seconds to induce a mild seizure, but because of the muscle relaxant, the only outward sign is a flickering of the eyelids. Usually, a series of 3 to 12 treatments is prescribed.

What is it used for?
ECT is potentially helpful only in certain circumstances and is usually used only when all other treatments have failed. Severe depression is the main indication, particularly in people who have suicidal tendencies or who have stopped eating and drinking. The treatment has also been shown to be useful in treating women who experience a psychotic illness following childbirth.

How does it work?
Experts are not exactly sure why ECT is effective. After a treatment session, however, the levels of some hormones and brain chemicals appear to increase. Whether these changes are relevant remains debatable.

Are there any adverse effects?
Serious side effects are rare and are usually attributable to a preexisting condition or the anesthetic. Most people have a headache, slight confusion, nausea or muscle pains. Short-term memory loss can result and may increase with each treatment, although available evidence so far points away from the development of long-term memory problems. There is ongoing concern and debate over the possibility that ECT might cause irreversible brain damage and memory loss. To date, there appears to be no evidence of obvious brain damage, although some experts believe that subtle cognitive changes may occur. Ultimately, these side effects must be balanced against the potentially life-threatening nature of severe depression.

Neurosurgical solutions

Neurosurgery is highly specialized and requires extreme precision; any damage to delicate nerve tissue could be devastating. Advances in medical technology have enabled surgeons to achieve this accuracy.

THE ROLE OF NEUROSURGERY
Neurosurgery has three main roles to play: to repair existing damage and make sure the vital blood supply to the brain is not affected, to prevent further damage to the tissue, and to cure some conditions.

Repairing damage
Neurosurgeons are often called upon to repair damage to the skull and backbone and to prevent further injury from occurring—in fact head injuries are among the most common conditions treated by the neurosurgical team. Most importantly, neurosurgeons must make sure that the blood supply to the brain is adequate—without a healthy supply of oxygenated blood, brain tissue dies within a few minutes and is not able to regenerate.

Preventing further injury
The skull is a tight compartment, and if the brain swells for any reason, for example if it is bruised or if there is a sudden bleed from a faulty blood vessel, surgeons must relieve the pressure quickly. This can be done with a life-saving operation to remove a small section of the skull.

Neurosurgery as a cure
In addition to dealing with trauma, the neurosurgical team treats long-term conditions, and many of the operations, such as for the removal of tumors, are planned well in advance. Persistent back problems, such as a slipped disk can sometimes be resolved with surgery. Neurosurgery is also an option for some physical deformities; for example, doctors can reconstruct the backbone using implants.

THE NEUROSURGICAL TEAM
As with any other medical specialty, the neurosurgical team consists of more than just a surgeon or two. A variety of health professionals contribute toward each patient's care and work together as a team, exchanging

information and ideas and discussing a treatment plan. The team is usually led by a senior doctor who will have specialized in this type of surgery for many years. In addition, there are several doctors on the team, each with a different level of experience. The neurosurgeons work closely with the nurses in the ward as well as with doctors from associated specialties, in particular radiologists, who play a role in identifying the exact location of damage and pathologists who determine the type of abnormality.

Some members of the team are primarily involved with recovery and rehabilitation following surgery. These include physical therapists, speech therapists, and occupational therapists, who will often begin to treat and advise patients before surgery so that each individual knows what to expect afterward and is well prepared. A day or two before the surgery, an anesthetist experienced in neurosurgical procedures assesses and examines the patient in readiness for a general anesthetic.

TOOLS OF THE TRADE

The first step in neurosurgery is gaining access to the brain, or the backbone or spinal cord. Usually, a section of skull needs to be removed during a procedure called a craniotomy (see page 125) before the affected part of the brain can be operated on—surgery on the spine may also involve taking away sections of the vertebrae. Specialist equipment therefore includes a high-speed drill and craniotome, which has an assortment of attachments that cut or drill through bone. Any fears that the drill might damage brain tissue are unfounded; a combination of the surgeon's skill and a safety mechanism on the instrument ensures that the drill can pass only through the depth of the skull. In addition, there is a tough protective layer called the dura between the skull and the brain tissue.

The importance of accuracy

Because of the delicate nature of neurosurgery and the vulnerability of brain tissue, the head must be carefully positioned for maximum stability. To this end, surgeons often insert small pins into the skull and attach them to a rigid arm connected to the operating table. The arm can then be adjusted to keep the head in a secure position. Most importantly, the surgeon must know exactly where in the brain he or she will be working and be able to reach that point with minimum upset to surrounding tissue. Any unnecessary interference with healthy brain tissue could have dramatic consequences, and surgeons do all in their power to avoid this.

Pinpointing the target

Images produced by plain X-rays, computed tomography scanning, and magnetic resonance imaging are examined carefully by the neuro-surgeons before the operation. It is during surgery, however, that accurate guidance is needed most. So that the surgeon can obtain a clear view, a microscope is often used to provide a magnified image of brain tissue. In addition, a technique called stereotaxy is particularly helpful for guiding the surgeon to the operating area via a specific safe route through the brain. Stereotaxy involves

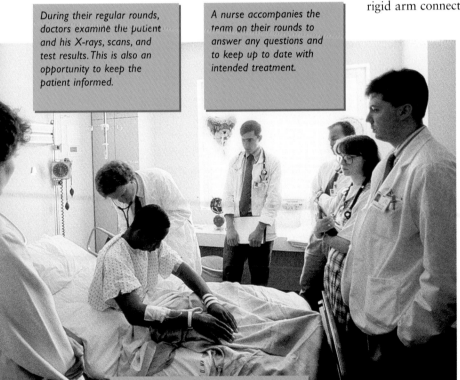

During their regular rounds, doctors examine the patient and his X-rays, scans, and test results. This is also an opportunity to keep the patient informed.

A nurse accompanies the team on their rounds to answer any questions and to keep up to date with intended treatment.

The physiotherapist is part of the neurosurgical team and has specialist skills in rehabilitation following surgery on the brain and spine.

Stereotaxy frame

This piece of equipment is placed over a patient's head before surgery and, in conjunction with brain scanning, provides an exact "grid reference" for a tumor (shown page 127, step 2).

placing a cage-like frame around the patient's head. The frame acts as a grid, and by scanning the brain with the frame in place and by using reference points and feeding information into a computer, the precise location of an abnormality is defined. Surgeons use this information to guide instruments to the target with minimal danger to healthy brain tissue.

A step forward from stereotaxy is the use of image guidance, in which a similar technique is used to obtain a three-dimensional image of the brain.

WHAT TO EXPECT BEFORE AND AFTER

The events preceding the operation very much depend on the reason for the surgery. In an emergency, doctors will probably want to carry out the operation as soon as

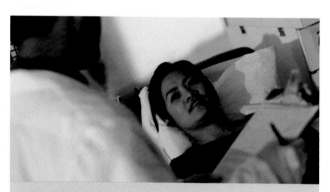

How long does it take?

These are only guidelines; the operation and recovery times for neurosurgery may vary among individuals.

BRAIN SURGERY	OPERATION TIME	RECOVERY TIME
Tumor removal	2 to 3 hours	5 days to 2 weeks
Craniotomy for a subarachnoid hemorrhage	3 to 4 hours	1 week to 3 months
SPINAL SURGERY	OPERATION TIME	RECOVERY TIME
Lumbar laminectomy	1 to 2 hours	4 days to 2 weeks
Microdiskectomy	Up to 1 hour	1 to 7 days
Cervical diskectomy	1 to 2 hours	4 days to 2 weeks

possible, and afterwards the patient may remember little or nothing at all about the preparation. If the operation is planned in advance, however, there should be plenty of opportunity to prepare a person for neurosurgery, both physically and psychologically.

The day of the operation

On the day of surgery, the patient will not be allowed to eat or drink for six hours before the operation to avoid going to the operating room with a full stomach. Contrary to popular belief, it is no longer necessary to shave the entire head for brain surgery. Instead, surgeons only shave a very small area of the scalp—just enough to make the incision—and they do this after the anesthetic has taken effect.

Asleep or awake?

Most neurosurgery is done under general anesthetia. In some cases, however, a local anesthetic into the scalp and an initial light anesthetic is all that is used. The patient can then be brought back to an awake state once a section of the skull has been removed and the surgeon has located the tumor in the brain. Neurosurgery under local anesthetic is known as an "awake craniotomy" and is carried out when it is important to be able to pinpoint precise areas of function, such as speech or movement, so the surgeon can be sure to avoid them.

Immediately after the operation

Following emergency surgery, a short time in the intensive care unit may be necessary. Here, one-on-one nursing and constant medical supervision mean that a patient's condition can be closely monitored for as long as necessary; transfer to a surgical ward takes place as soon as a patient is stable.

Going home

Rehabilitation procedures and recovery times depend on the extent of the surgery; see the chart on the left for some example recovery times. As a rule, the more fit a person is before the operation, the quicker he or she will recover. Whatever the situation, however, once a person is fully recovered from the anesthetic, the multidisciplinary team swings into action to get each individual fit to go home as soon as possible.

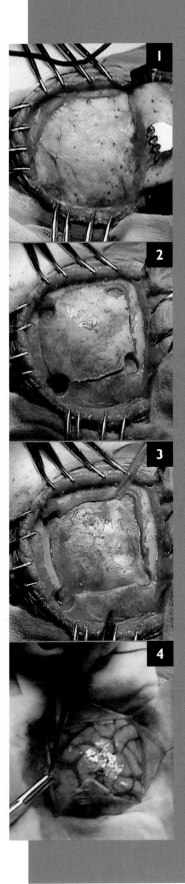

Craniotomy—exposing the brain for surgery

1 Once the patient is anesthetised, a small area of the scalp is shaved and swabbed with a cleaning fluid. The surgeon makes an incision through the skin with a scalpel. The scalp has an abundant blood supply, so any bleeding vessels are secured with clips. The skin is then pulled back with retractors.

2 The surgeon uses a special drill to make holes at selected points in the skull. Using a cutting instrument or a high-speed drill, the surgeon isolates the bone flap by cutting between the holes.

3 The flap is lifted off the brain using either a pair of forceps or an instrument called an elevator, to reveal the dura (the tough membrane surrounding the brain) underneath.

4 The dura is lifted upward with a sharp hook, cut with scissors, and peeled back—the brain is now exposed.

Once the surgery is complete, the dura is stitched back together and the bony skull flap is replaced and secured with strong stitches.

SURGICAL PROCEDURES

For most types of brain surgery, whether an emergency or a routine operation, a craniotomy is the first step—this is the term for the removal of a part of the skull, which allows further surgery to take place. At the end of the operation, the skull section is usually secured back into position with strong stitches. If the operation is on the spine, a skin incision is usually all that is necessary.

Once inside the skull . . .

Emergency neurosurgery to reduce the pressure in the skull might be necessary following a head injury or bleeding in the brain. In these cases, a craniotomy is often carried out as soon as possible to remove a blood clot that is exerting pressure on the brain. If the bleeding is because of a ruptured artery, called a subarachnoid hemorrhage, urgent measures may be necessary to find the affected artery and prevent further bleeding.

Routine surgery includes the removal of various types of brain tumor, both malignant and benign. Sometimes treatment for a brain tumor will combine radiotherapy, chemotherapy and surgery. Neurosurgeons also routinely treat hydrocephalus, a condition in which there is too much fluid in the brain. A fine drainage tube is inserted into the fluid-producing cavities of the brain and passed down the body to the abdomen or chest.

A rare type of neurosurgery is carried out in some people with Parkinson's disease, epilepsy, or obsessive–compulsive disorder to remove or destroy the particular part of the brain causing the problem. This surgery is carried out only in certain circumstances, however, after all other treatment has failed.

Removing a brain tumor

Now that surgeons have perfected the techniques to gain access to the brain, by removing part of the skull, they can perform complex operations to remove brain tumors, particularly benign ones, with a high rate of success.

The brain sits within a nonexpandable box—the skull. Because of the snug fit, any extra volume such as a growth within the skull can increase the internal pressure, and compress and damage the delicate brain tissue. Therefore, even benign (noncancerous) brain tumours can have serious consequences, particularly if vital areas of the brain are affected, such as those controlling vision, speech, or movement. Ideally, a benign tumor should be removed, although there are some instances when this is not possible.

What used to be lengthy, complex and risky surgery is today much more routine—removal of a benign brain tumor can often take less than three hours. Even the makeup of the tumor can be determined on the spot by a pathologist, who is often able to examine a sample of tissue and confirm the diagnosis while the surgeon is still operating.

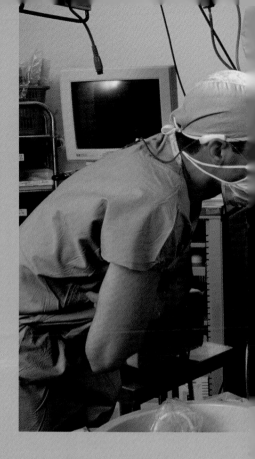

Mapping the brain for surgical accuracy

Advances in scanning techniques and high-tech methods of locating the position of a tumor have made neurosurgery safer, more accurate, and often 100 percent successful. Although the neurosurgeon will have studied scans closely before surgery, these images will also be displayed prominently in the operating room so they can be viewed at any time during the operation (below). This magnetic resonance imaging scan (right) shows a tumor in the left side of the brain.

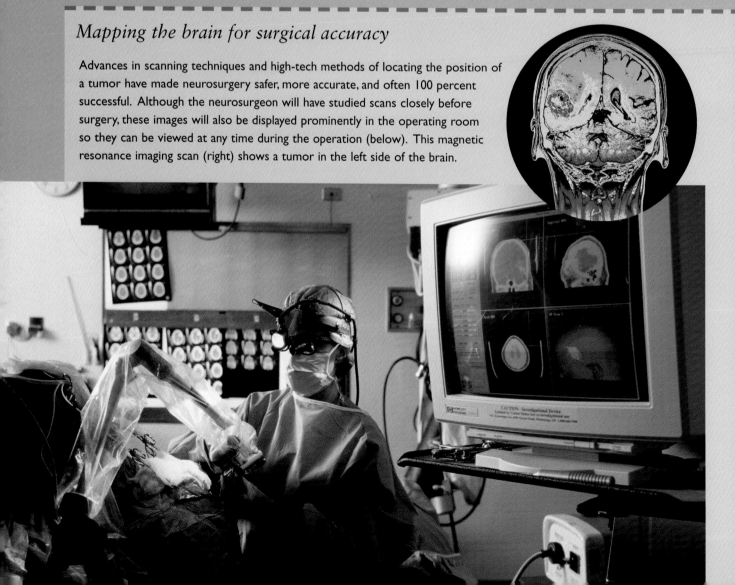

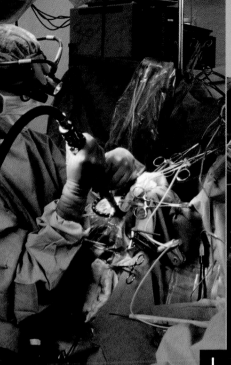

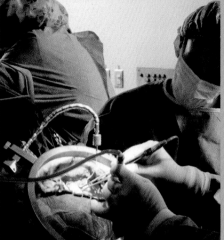

1 2

The surgical procedure

1 First, using a high-speed drill and craniotome, the surgeon performs a craniotomy (see page 125) to remove a section of the skull and gain access to the brain. If the tumor is hidden in a groove, the brain is gently retracted and the covering membranes (dura) are cut away to expose the tumor.

2 Using a microscope, the surgeon carefully cuts away the edge of the tumor from the surrounding brain tissue with highly engineered microinstruments.

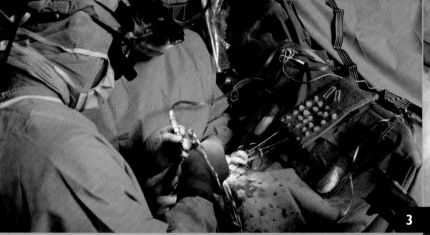

3 4

3 The tumor, like the brain, may have a rich blood supply so the blood vessels must be sealed using electrocoagulation forceps, which seal the bleeding point using an electric current. Surgeons can also control bleeding with special gauze made from a substance that encourages blood to clot.

4 The surgeon removes the tumor by working all the way around it to separate it from the brain. For a large tumor, the center is often removed first, keeping clear of the brain tissue itself—a process called debulking.

5 After the tumor is removed, the surgeon irrigates the brain with warm saline to clean the area and to keep it moist. The tissue is carefully inspected for bleeding areas, and any bleeding vessels are sealed. The surgeon then closes the area: Brain tissue and then the skull and scalp flaps are replaced and secured with sutures.

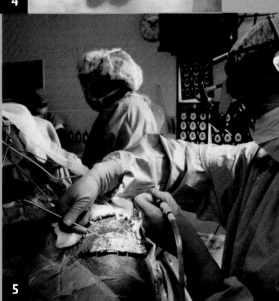

5

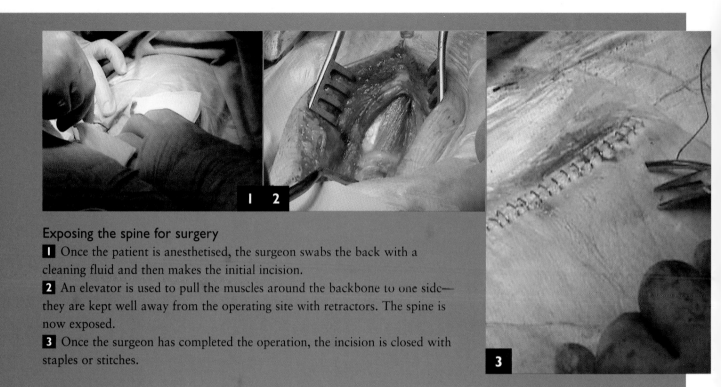

Exposing the spine for surgery
1 Once the patient is anesthetised, the surgeon swabs the back with a cleaning fluid and then makes the initial incision.
2 An elevator is used to pull the muscles around the backbone to one side—they are kept well away from the operating site with retractors. The spine is now exposed.
3 Once the surgeon has completed the operation, the incision is closed with staples or stitches.

SPINAL SURGERY

Spinal surgery includes operations on the backbones (vertebrae), spinal cord, nerve roots and muscles, and ligaments. The majority of operations on the spine are performed to improve wear and tear, but spinal surgery may also be necessary after an accident. Occasionally, surgeons operate to remove a tumor growing on the spinal cord.

The spinal cord is the main pathway for nerves passing between the brain and the rest of the body, so the main concern for surgeons is to protect the cord and to prevent further damage from occurring.

Treating "wear and tear"

Deteriorating bones is one of the hazards of aging, and the backbone is particularly vulnerable to wear and tear. Thickening in the lamina of the vertebrae—the hard knobs you can feel down your back—can cause abnormal pressure on the spinal cord and can lead to unpleasant symptoms. During an operation called a laminectomy, surgeons can trim away the excess bone and relieve the pressure on the spine.

Other commonly performed operations are a lumbar microdiskectomy and cervical diskectomy, both of which repair a "slipped disc." A disk is the cartilaginous tissue between the vertebrae and commonly ruptures as a result of lifting a heavy load incorrectly. The usual consequences of a slipped disk are restricted mobility and pain, and although sometimes rest is enough to resolve the symptoms, in severe cases surgery may be necessary.

Using a microscope for a clear view, the surgeon makes a small incision, either in the back or in the neck (depending on the level of the injury), and removes part of the disk. As the disks are needed to act as buffers between the vertebrae, only the fragment that has slipped is removed, leaving the remaining disk tissue in place.

Surgery after trauma

If the spine is injured during trauma, for example as the result of a fractured backbone, the role of the neurosurgeon is to stabilize the spine and relieve any pressure, so that no further damage is sustained. Any injury to the spinal cord is irreversible—a damaged spinal cord cannot be repaired. If the damage is severe, the spine can be stabilized using metal implants or plates.

Spinal tumours

Very occasionally, a rare spinal tumor can press on the spinal cord and cause problems. In these cases, the surgeon may decide to remove the tumor.

Recovering from a stroke

The mention of stroke conjures up images of long-term illness, paralysis, even death, and yet the real picture is often very different. With today's emphasis on rehabilitation, many people who have had a stroke regain their independence and return to live at home.

WHAT IS A STROKE?

A stroke occurs when part of the brain is deprived of oxygen, either by a blockage in an artery or bleeding in the brain tissue itself. The resulting symptoms depend on the area affected and the severity of the damage.

The most common symptoms of a stroke are weakness or paralysis of one side of the body, altered body sensation, partial loss of the field of vision and either difficulties with speech and language (if the stroke has occurred in the left side of the brain) or problems with visual and spatial awareness (if the stroke has affected the right side of the brain). Some people also have psychological symptoms such as loss of memory, and changes in behavior and emotional reactions.

The important thing to remember is that for most people the initial problems improve. In the first few days, however, symptoms such as partial paralysis and slurred speech can be frightening for all concerned. The first priority is for the doctors to make a clear diagnosis and to prevent, as far as possible, any further damage to the brain. Rehabilitation can begin only once the medical problems are under control.

HOW LONG DOES RECOVERY TAKE?

As with all physical injury, recovery depends on the severity of the stroke. The brain has an amazing ability to adapt and recover—a phenomenon that experts still do not fully understand—and the outlook for stroke victims is far better than most people imagine. In fact, the majority of the 8 in 10 patients who survive a stroke return home, especially if a rehabilitation program is begun as soon as possible.

As a general rule, physical recovery occurs in the same sequence as a young child learning to move. At first, paralysis of one side of the body can prevent a person from even rolling over in bed. In much the same way as a baby learns to sit, to stand, and eventually to progress to walking, a stroke victim may have to relearn those stages. At times this can be slow and frustrating, particularly if there are additional language or speech problems. With the support of healthcare professionals, however, many skills can be regained within months of the stroke. Even if the ability to walk does not completely return, standing with help or with a walker is often possible.

THE REHABILITATION TEAM

Because stroke can affect so many aspects of a person's life, rehabilitation is coordinated by a team of healthcare professionals. Family members and friends are also closely involved in rehabilitation. Before planning a program, the team will need to know the exact nature of the person's disabilities and capabilities, which can vary

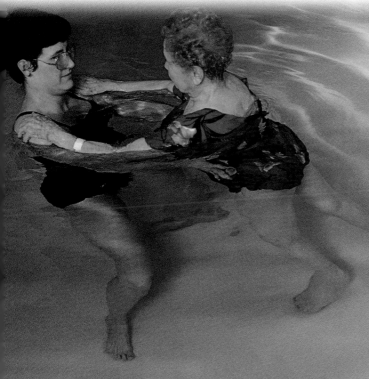

Keeping as active as possible
After a stroke, weak and stiff limbs can benefit enormously from regular sessions in a hydrotherapy pool with a physical therapist. Hydrotherapy is usually just part of a tailor-made rehabilitation program to help regain skills.

immensely. In some cases, for example, the symptoms are so mild that admission to a hospital is not necessary and treatment is provided in the community, whereas in others, a lengthy stay in a hospital may be necessary.

Who are the team members?

Contact with nurses and doctors occurs mainly in a hospital, where the priorities are focused on treating the cause of the stroke, making sure the patient is comfortable, and providing support and advice for the whole family. The rest of the team will be involved in the first instance in the hospital but will continue to provide support at home.

- A physical therapist becomes involved from an early stage, ensuring good positioning in bed and in a chair before prescribing exercise to regain motor skills, such as balance and coordination, which are necessary for walking.
- An occupational therapist assists with physical functions such as the ability to dress and eat, as well as leisure activities and a return to work, if applicable. The therapist also makes sure that, if possible, appropriate equipment is installed in the home before discharge.
- Early in rehabilitation, a speech and language therapist becomes involved and not only helps a patient with communication challenges but also provides advice if the ability to swallow is affected.
- As with any chronic illness, many people lose their appetite; a dietitian can assess individual needs.
- Finally, a social worker may become involved, particularly when the time approaches to return home and begin regaining as normal a lifestyle as possible.

Is depression inevitable after stroke?

It is absolutely normal to feel down in the dumps following a stroke—physical discomfort, fear of the future, and a feeling of uselessness can all contribute to quite severe depression in many people. The most important thing is not to keep concerns bottled up. There is enough to think about just concentrating on returning to life outside the hospital.

Often, simply expressing fears to family and friends or a member of the rehabilitation team is enough. If, however, the symptoms of depression become worse or don't seem to be improving, a visit to your doctor is probably advisable. He or she may well prescribe antidepressant pills until the initial pressures of coping with a new life begin to lessen.

ASK THE EXPERT

WHAT DOES THE FUTURE HOLD?

Virtually all patients will have some remaining disability, but this may range from an occasional difficulty in remembering a word to completely losing the ability to walk. Approaches to rehabilitation vary immensely, but no single technique is more effective than another. The most important factor is that goals that have been mutually agreed upon by the patient, the family, and the rehabilitation team, are eventually reached.

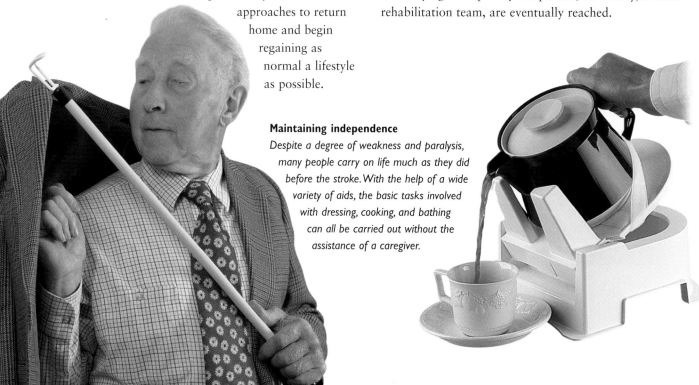

Maintaining independence
Despite a degree of weakness and paralysis, many people carry on life much as they did before the stroke. With the help of a wide variety of aids, the basic tasks involved with dressing, cooking, and bathing can all be carried out without the assistance of a caregiver.

A TO Z

OF DISEASES AND DISORDERS

This section provides information on the main illnesses and medical conditions that can affect the brain and central nervous system. The entries are arranged alphabetically and give the following information for each condition:

What are the causes?

What are the symptoms?

How is it diagnosed?

What are the treatment options?

What is the outlook?

How can it be prevented or minimized?

ABSCESS IN THE BRAIN
A rare condition in which an infection causes a collection of pus to build up in the brain.

The brain is well protected from the outside world by the skull, so an abscess develops usually because infection has spread from nearby organs or tissues, such as the sinuses, ears, or a tooth. Sometimes, however, infectious organisms find a direct route into brain tissue following a head injury. Occasionally, an abscess is due to infection that travels from elsewhere in the body, for example, the lungs.

What are the symptoms?
Headache, frequently worse in the morning, along with nausea and vomiting are usually the first signs of a brain abscess, but exact symptoms depend on the part of the brain affected. If, for example, the abscess is in the area of the brain that controls movement, weakness of the arms and legs may develop. Likewise, difficulty in speaking, understanding, or both occur if the abscess affects the speech centers. A third of people with an abscess will have seizures, and some will develop a fever because of the infection.

How is it diagnosed?
The only way to accurately diagnose an abscess is to obtain a clear picture of the brain. Brain imaging techniques, such as computed tomography scanning (p. 106) or magnetic resonance imaging (p. 108), can highlight an abscess as a distinctive ring-shaped abnormality, usually with some swelling in the surrounding tissue. Imaging can also help to identify the source of the infection.

What are the treatment options?
Generally, a brain abscess requires treatment by a neuro-surgeon. The exact operation depends on the location of the abscess, but often a small hole is made in the skull and the fluid in the abscess is drained. A sample of abscess fluid is examined under a microscope, and once the pathogen is identified, an appropriate antibiotic is prescribed, usually for a period of several weeks.

What is the outlook?
A brain abscess is usually a very serious condition requiring at least a few weeks treatment in a hospital; in some cases, it can be life threatening. Many people recover completely, but about a third to half continue to have long-term difficulties, which could include weakness of a limb, seizures, and speech disorders.

ADDICTION AND WITHDRAWAL
A behavior is characterized as "addictive" when its use is "excessive" and its purpose is to satisfy an "appetite." Removing the source of the addiction creates withdrawal as the body craves what it is used to.

Addiction can apply to the consumption of drugs or alcohol or to behaviors such as gambling or stealing. Doctors classify drug use as experimental (trying out a few times), recreational (using regularly within social groups), or dependent (when there are psychological, medical, and social consequences of its use and cessation). Dependency always includes a compulsion to take the drug on a continuous or periodic basis in order to experience its effects and sometimes to avoid the discomfort of its absence. Psychological features are restlessness and craving, whereas biological features include tolerance and withdrawal symptoms. Developing tolerance means that the body has adjusted to the drug and more is needed each time to produce the same effects.

What are the causes?
The reasons for addiction and dependence on, for example, a drug are biological, psychological, and social. Several mechanisms have been explored to understand how tolerance develops biologically. One theory is that brain cells adapt to a drug so that if the drug is no longer taken, the cells cannot function alone and withdrawal symptoms occur.

If something we do produces pleasant effects or helps reduce unpleasant effects, we are more likely to repeat it. This applies to addictions—the very effects of the act reinforce its use. Although there is no evidence of an "addictive personality," individual characteristics such as the experience of an unhappy childhood are common. Important social factors are linked to availability, cultural acceptance, and social pressures to indulge.

How is it diagnosed?
Addiction can be identified by several criteria:
- The person feels a craving or compulsion to take the substance or carry on the behavior.
- There is evidence of increasing tolerance and salience when using the behavior, or seeking and taking the substance, takes priority in the person's life.
- Stereotyping occurs—for example, the person takes only a preferred drink or specific brand of cigarette.
- There are repeated withdrawal symptoms when the behavior or drug is stopped.

- There is rapid reuse after a period of abstinence.
- Withdrawal symptoms are relieved or avoided by using the behavior or substance.

Most but not all of these criteria are important to establish a diagnosis of addiction or dependence syndrome. The most important features are the compulsion, salience, lack of control over the behavior, and distress when stopping.

What are the treatment options?
Treatment is dependent on the addiction and the individual factors that led to it. Most treatment programs combine slow withdrawal (detoxification) with psychological and social support, or, in the case of behavioral problems, the instigation of appropriate therapy. Rehabilitation is crucial to reestablish the individual within a new social network away from the cause of the addiction and to enable a gradual return to work and everyday life.

AIDS-RELATED DISORDERS
Conditions of the nervous system that arise because of the presence of the human immunodeficiency virus (HIV). Any one of these conditions usually indicates that a person has acquired immunodeficiency syndrome (AIDS).

HIV targets the body's immune system. In many people, the virus weakens the system so much that it becomes unable to defend itself against "opportunistic" infections and rare cancers, which can infect the brain and spinal cord.

What are the causes?
Pathogenic organisms can invade the brain to cause meningitis, viral encephalitis, or a brain abscess. In addition, rare cancers can develop in the brain. The following conditions specifically affect people whose immune systems are faulty:
- A rare and serious form of meningitis, caused by a fungus called *Cryptococcus*
- A potentially fatal inflammation in the brain—encephalitis—caused by the *Toxoplasma* parasite
- Severe viral encephalitis due to the herpes simplex virus—the virus that causes cold sores
- Inflammation in the brain caused by the cytomegalovirus
- A rare brain cancer called primary cerebral lymphoma

In addition to these rare, potentially fatal infections of the brain, HIV can directly damage the nervous system. Depending on the area affected, the patient may show signs of dementia, weakness in the legs, and pain and numbness in the feet.

How is it diagnosed?
In a person who is not known to be HIV positive, developing any one of these conditions may be the first indication of AIDS, so a test may be done to confirm HIV status. If a person is known to be infected with HIV, the individual symptoms will give a clue to which part of the nervous system is affected. Numerous tests will be necessary to get a diagnosis, such as blood tests (p. 101) to look for evidence of infection, or a spinal tap (p. 103) and computed tomography scanning (p. 106) or magnetic resonance imaging (p. 108) of the brain to check for the presence of a tumor or abnormal swelling. Occasionally a brain biopsy (p. 112) may be necessary to distinguish a tumor from a brain abscess.

What are the treatment options?
Combinations of drugs can slow down the decline in the immune system by reducing the rate at which HIV replicates in the body. This can help the immune system to prevent rare infections and cancers from developing. These drugs can also improve some of the neurological symptoms, such as dementia, although they can themselves cause adverse effects, such as nerve pain in the limbs. Most complications can be treated with appropriate drugs, but because the conditions are often so serious, even prompt and aggressive treatment is not always successful. Steroids can improve primary cerebral lymphoma by reducing swelling in the brain. Radiation and chemotherapy can slow the growth of a tumor, but they cannot cure the condition.

ALCOHOLISM
The term refers to any alcohol-related disorder, but in essence it means alcohol dependence and the adverse health and social consequences of excessive drinking.

The effects of alcohol vary from person to person and depend on the quantity consumed. Alcohol abuse carries a number of neurological and psychiatric implications.

What are the causes?
When a person drinks a constantly high level of alcohol, the body develops a physical dependence on it; this means that when the person stops drinking he or she experiences withdrawal symptoms and starts to crave another drink. Although social acceptance and the availability of alcohol has some influence on the pattern of alcohol-related disorders, the development of alcohol dependence

In 1999, alcohol was responsible for more than 1.3 million hospital visits in the United States. It cost $167 billion per year in medical care, criminal justice costs, damages, and lost earnings.

syndrome is due to interacting genetic, psychological, and social factors. The genetic component is probably related to personality type as well as the level of alcohol required to induce biological dependence. There is no "alcoholic personality," and in some people the cause of dependence can be more cogently linked to low self-esteem or current life difficulties. Heavier drinking is more commonly associated with men but is increasing in women. It is also particularly prevalent in certain occupations: those involved with the sale and manufacture of alcohol, company directors, journalists, entertainers, and doctors.

What are the symptoms?
The main symptoms of alcohol dependence syndrome are
- Increased tolerance to alcohol
- Repeated withdrawal symptoms and avoidance or relief of withdrawal symptoms by drinking
- Awareness of the compulsion to drink
- Rapid return to drinking following attempts to stop
- Drinking and drink-seeking behavior taking precedence in the person's life
- Restricting drinking to specific types of drink

How is it diagnosed?
Apart from the presence of the symptoms listed above, a diagnosis is made when the physical complications of alcohol abuse become apparent through liver damage, gastrointestinal complications, or withdrawal symptoms.

What are the treatment options?
Most treatment programs offer detoxification with psychological and social support. This may require inpatient admission to a therapeutic program, but can also be done as an outpatient. Rehabilitation is important to reestablish the individual within a new social network away from the culture of alcohol and gradually return them to work and everyday life. Rehabilitation also includes psychotherapy and self-help group work.

What is the outlook?
Successful treatment is often linked to motivation; those people who have enough willpower, or a strong enough reason to commit to giving up alcohol, can live an alcohol-free life. But success also depends on the complexity of the causes for each individual.

ALZHEIMER'S DISEASE
see Dementia (p. 139)

AMNESIA
A person with amnesia has difficulty both in recalling memories and in creating new ones.

Usually we associate memory loss with aging, and indeed amnesia does often occur in people with Alzheimer's disease and other types of dementias. There are, however, other conditions that cause memory loss, including
- Head injury
- Stroke
- Viral infection of the brain, known as encephalitis
- Wernicke–Korsakoff syndrome—a severe deficiency of vitamin B (thiamine) that affects alcoholics

One type of amnesia—transient global amnesia—is an unusual condition that tends to affect middle-aged and elderly people. A person will suddenly, and for no reason, suffer complete memory loss lasting for up to eight hours. Although people recover completely, they are unable to recall anything that happened during the attack. Doctors are unsure of the cause of transient global amnesia, but it is now thought to be related to migraine (p. 145).

What are the symptoms?
In addition to memory loss, a person with amnesia often asks questions over and over again. Family or friends will describe a sudden onset of odd behavior with repetitive questioning and anxiety.

How is it diagnosed?
In many people, amnesia is a symptom itself rather than an isolated condition. The diagnostic process, therefore, tends to center around the disorder causing the amnesia. For example, if a stroke or head injury is suspected, the doctor will arrange an X-ray (p. 104) or brain scan (p. 106), and blood tests (p. 101); a history of alcohol abuse can confirm a diagnosis of Wernicke–Korsakoff syndrome.

What are the treatment options?
If memory does not return following treatment for any underlying disorder, memory aids such as structuring the daily routine and using lists, reminder notes, and pager systems can help a person to live a normal life. For people with severe amnesia, however, long-term care and supervision may be necessary to ensure their safety.

ANXIETY AND PANIC ATTACKS
An extreme form of anxiety that becomes a neurosis. Extreme, unpredictable bouts of anxiety are called panic attacks.

Anxiety is a normal and useful feeling. Its original biological function was to signal potential harm from predators and trigger the fight-or-flight response. Anxiety becomes a problem when the feelings are out of proportion with the circumstances in either intensity or duration. Mild anxiety helps us to focus on the task required, but excessive amounts can paralyze us and ruin our performance.

What are the causes?
A tendency toward anxiety or being an "excessive worrier" seems to be partly inherited and becomes apparent during stressful times. Panic attacks can have several causes:
• An overactive thyroid gland
• Certain types of medication
• Consuming too many caffeinated drinks
• Taking illicit drugs, such as amphetamines or Ecstasy
Excessive anxiety or panic attacks also occur when people are depressed or have other psychiatric conditions such as posttraumatic stress disorder or a phobia.

What are the symptoms?
An anxiety disorder is characterized by
• Worrying thoughts that cannot be controlled
• Feeling tired, tense, and irritable
• Restlessness and inability to concentrate
There are also physical symptoms, including an irregular heart beat, sweating and diarrhea, and muscle tension. These symptoms will occur on most days and prevent the person from carrying out everyday activities.

How is it diagnosed?
Underlying physiological causes of excessive anxiety or panic attacks must be ruled out before a psychological problem can be established. This also
applies to determining if the anxiety symptoms are part of another psychiatric disorder, in particular depression or a phobia. A true panic attack will consist of several of the physical symptoms listed above with a feeling of intense fear occurring at the same time. A doctor usually makes the diagnosis based on the medical history and physical examination (p. 98).

Physical sensations of anxiety, such as "butterflies in the stomach," trembling hands, or wobbly legs, are all quite normal.

HAVING A PANIC ATTACK

As far as I was concerned, I was dying. It started with a racing feeling and an ache in my chest, and pretty quickly I was fighting for breath.

My whole body was shaking and dripping with sweat. My hands and legs had pins and needles—I couldn't keep still. The feeling of giddiness and nausea was overwhelming, and I honestly thought I was losing control. The first attack lasted for about ten minutes, but since then I've had episodes that lasted for hours.

Afterwards, my doctor diagnosed an anxiety disorder— she advised therapy and prescribed medication, which has really helped. Apparently, the symptoms are caused by an extra spurt of particular hormones called epinephrine and norepinephrine. They don't know the reason for this, but anxiety disorders can run in families. Severe stress and a difficult childhood can also contribute.

What are the treatment options?
Anxiety or panic attacks that have underlying psychological causes such as phobias and depression will usually resolve as those disorders are treated. A secondary problem can develop if someone who experiences high levels of anxiety or panic begins to self-medicate using drugs or, particularly, alcohol. A variety of approaches can help, including self-help groups, general counseling, relaxation techniques, and stress management. More specific treatments include medication and psychotherapy. Drugs for anxiety (p. 117) should only be part of the treatment package. Valium-like substances are for short-term use only because of their addictive qualities.

Psychotherapy is widely practiced and can take the form of individual or group therapy. Behavioral techniques and cognitive behavior therapy have been established as two of the best treatments. A very condensed and simplistic explanation of these approaches would be this: the therapist works with the anxious person to examine the underlying belief systems and tries to elicit the thoughts that occur before a panic starts, which may therefore precipitate or worsen an attack.

CEREBRAL PALSY
A condition in which the part of the brain controlling movement and posture does not develop properly.

Cerebral palsy is a group of symptoms caused by brain damage sustained during pregnancy or childbirth. For most cases, there is no easily identifiable cause. Some infections, however, such as rubella or cytomegalovirus can damage the delicate tissues of a baby's brain *in utero* if the infection is contracted by the mother during pregnancy. Rarely, cerebral palsy can result from a difficult birth if a baby is starved of vital oxygen. After birth, the condition usually affects only premature babies, whose immature brains are more vulnerable to damage from infection or poor blood supply. Occasionally, however, a child develops cerebral palsy after a severe case of meningitis or a head injury.

What are the symptoms?
The degree to which cerebral palsy affects individuals varies enormously, and symptoms range from very mild to severely disabling. Children with cerebral palsy are not necessarily affected in terms of learning ability and often have normal intelligence. A baby with cerebral palsy might not be diagnosed until the age of six months, when he or she should begin to move independently. The symptoms become more obvious with time as the child does not achieve developmental milestones. Problems with movement (the most affected function) can be apparent in many ways, and a child may have some or all of the following:
• Poor coordination of movement, along with stiff muscles
• An unsteady walk with balancing difficulties
• Uncontrollable or involuntary movements
• Problems with speech and swallowing

How is it diagnosed?
A doctor will usually diagnose cerebral palsy on the basis of its quite distinctive symptoms. The main concern for the family is a delay in the diagnosis and the resulting shock once symptoms become obvious. Computed tomography scanning (p. 106) or magnetic resonance imaging (p. 108) of the brain is performed to identify any obvious brain damage.

What are the treatment options?
Once brain tissue has been damaged it cannot be repaired, so treatment focuses more on encouraging independence than on a cure. Regular exercise can help to keep limbs supple, and a physcal therapist can work with a child to improve mobility and balance. Mildly affected children can attend school and integrate well with other children. Severely affected children (who may have very limited mobility and learning ability) may need full-time care in a special center, although parental care at home is possible. As with any disability, there is a network of specialist support available on which families can draw if they need to.

What is the outlook?
Many people with cerebral palsy have a normal lifespan with little or no illness during that time. A few children, however, have persistent chest infections because they cannot cough properly, and these may prove fatal.

COMA AND BRAIN DEATH
Coma is an altered level of consciousness causing a reduced response to stimuli. In brain death, the brainstem no longer functions and cannot sustain life.

Although brain death is sometimes the outcome of a coma, the two conditions have one very important difference: A person can recover from a coma and live a normal life, but someone with brain death is technically dead and will not recover. Brain death is an emotive diagnosis, not least because as long as life support continues, and breathing is carried out by a machine, none of the outward signs of death are present. Thus, accepting that brain death has occurred can be extremely difficult.

What is a persistent vegetative state?

People in a persistent vegetative state are completely unaware of their surroundings and do not respond to any stimulus at all. Despite this, they still appear to have routine sleep patterns and open and close their eyes normally. The automatic functions of the body, such as breathing, continue to work so that a life-support system is not necessary, although artificial feeding is required to avoid dehydration and starvation.

Although there is still controversy about persistent vegetative state, experts generally believe that recovery is not possible, although an affected person can live for years or even decades with full nursing care.

ASK THE EXPERT

What are the causes?

Any disease or injury that affects brain function can ultimately cause coma. Brain death occurs when the damage is so severe that the part of the brain called the brainstem, which is responsible for automatic body functions such as breathing, completely stops functioning. Causes of damage include

- Head injuries due to physical trauma
- Stroke and brain hemorrhage
- Hydrocephalus (water on the brain)
- An overdose of drugs or alcohol
- Uncontrolled diabetes mellitus
- Conditions that cause imbalances in the body, such as kidney failure and cirrhosis of the liver
- A severe continuous epileptic seizure (*status epilepticus*)
- Meningitis or encephalitis (brain inflammation)
- Severe infections (especially in the elderly)

What are the symptoms?

A person in a coma appears to be in deep sleep and does not usually respond to any outside stimulus. There are, however, varying degrees of coma, and in some cases a person will stir when spoken to or touched. Doctors use a scale called the Glasgow Coma Scale to assess how deeply unconscious a person is. In cases of brain death, the person is unable to breathe without life support, and cannot speak or make any purposeful movement.

How is it diagnosed?

In some situations, the cause of a coma may be self-evident, for example if a person has sustained a head injury. In others, doctors may find it more difficult to establish a cause. Knowing what happened in the period before the coma developed is extremely important, as is a medical examination. The doctor will usually request blood tests (p. 101), computed tomography scanning (p. 106) or magnetic resonance imaging (p. 108) of the brain, and an electroencephalogram (p. 111). If the doctor suspects meningitis or encephalitis, a spinal tap (p. 103) may be performed to take a sample of cerebrospinal fluid, which can then be examined for any signs of infection.

A diagnosis of brain death has to be 100 percent certain, because once doctors are sure of the diagnosis, decisions about continuation of life support have to be made. Two experienced senior doctors are required to carry out the series of tests necessary to diagnose brainstem death. Each of these tests checks the function of a particular nerve arising from the brainstem. If none of the nerves is

Should organ donation be automatic?

Donating your kidneys, heart, and lungs upon your death can be life-saving to other patients, and the corneas of your eyes could restore sight to a blind person. In the United Kingdom, waiting lists for transplants are steadily growing and only a small percentage of the population carry signed donor cards indicating a wish to donate their organs. Furthermore, up to 1 in 4 people who carry cards—the "opt in" system—have their wishes contradicted after death by family members, who for personal reasons object to donation. In the United States, donors either carry a donor card or include information on their drivers' licenses, another "opt-in" system. Donors are encouraged to make family members aware of their decision to donate. France, Belgium, and Austria have passed laws that assume everyone is willing to donate organs unless they specifically "opt out." This automatic system provides a greater number of potential transplant donors has the power to reduce waiting lists and save lives.

functioning and the affected person cannot breathe without a ventilator, it is clear that the brainstem is irreversibly damaged and that brain death has taken place.

What are the treatment options?

Whatever the cause, a person in a coma always needs emergency treatment, usually in an intensive care unit. In cases of head injury and bleeding, life-saving emergency surgery (p. 122) may be needed to relieve the pressure in the brain. Once doctors have diagnosed the condition causing the coma, they will be able to give appropriate treatment. For example, a person with uncontrolled diabetes can be stabilized either by giving insulin or by giving extra sugar.

What is the outcome?

For people in a coma, there are four potential outcomes: they may recover consciousness; they may enter a persistent vegetative state; they may suffer brain death; or the effects of the illness that caused the coma may prove fatal. To some extent, the outcome depends on how much and which areas of the brain are damaged, and even after a recovery, some people are left with a degree of disability.

CREUTZFELDT–JAKOB DISEASE
A rare infection of the brain that results in a form of progressive dementia.

CJD affects about one person in a million in the United States each year.

Creutzfeldt–Jakob disease (CJD) is incredibly rare, and yet the disease is one of the most talked about medical conditions today, mainly as a result of publicity surrounding new variant CJD. This form of the disease was first reported in the United Kingdom in 1995 and differs from classical CJD, which doctors were already aware of, in that it tends to affect young people and the symptoms take longer to develop.

What are the causes?
The damage from CJD is caused by the build-up of an infectious protein, called a prion, in brain tissue. In classical CJD, the reason is usually unknown, but the infection is occasionally transmitted through a medical procedure, such as a corneal graft or injection of growth hormone. Even more rarely, CJD is inherited from a parent with an abnormal gene.

Experts now believe that new variant CJD is caused by eating beef products infected with bovine spongiform encephalopathy (BSE), widely referred to as mad cow disease. This disease was found in British cattle in the 1980s and was probably caused by contaminated cattle feed, produced from carcasses of other animals. Recent research has shown that the same prion type that causes BSE in cattle also causes new variant CJD in humans and differs from the prion strains of classical CJD.

What are the symptoms?
How quickly symptoms develop depends on the type of CJD. Classical CJD is a rapidly progressive illness and is usually fatal within six months. A combination of the following symptoms develops over a few months:
• Irritability and personality change
• Poor memory and dementia
• Unsteadiness walking
• Jerking of the limbs (sometimes seizures)
• Visual symptoms and hallucinations
• Incontinence
In new variant CJD, symptoms are often vague at first, with a combination of
• Depression, irritability, and insomnia
• Discomfort or tingling in the face or limbs
After several months, symptoms similar to those of classical CJD develop. The illness usually lasts for about one to two years, after which time it is fatal.

How is it diagnosed?
As yet, there is no specific test available for CJD. The doctor may suspect CJD from a description of the onset of the illness, the symptoms, and a physical examination and confirm the diagnosis with the following tests.

An electroencephalogram of the electrical activity in the brain (p. 111) will often show specific abnormalities in CJD cases. Magnetic resonance imaging (p. 108) or computed tomography scanning (p. 106) is usually performed to exclude other possible causes of dementia. A spinal tap (p. 103) may be done to check for substances in the cerebrospinal fluid that indicate CJD. Doctors may take a tissue sample (p. 112), because recent research has proved that the prion protein can be present in the tonsils of people with new variant CJD. Blood samples (p. 101) may be taken to look for genetic abnormalities.

What are the treatment options?
There is no effective treatment for CJD at present, so care focuses on controlling the unpleasant symptoms of the disease, such as depression and jerking limbs.

How can it be prevented or minimized?
In families with inherited CJD, genetic counseling may be helpful for family members who may be at risk, especially if they are considering having children. Only central nervous system tissue has been shown to be infectious in classical CJD, so it is unlikely that the infection will be spread from

Will there be a CJD epidemic?

TALKING POINT

As of April 2002, 117 people in Britain had been diagnosed with new variant CJD. The first cases were diagnosed 10 years after the beginning of the BSE (mad cow disease) epidemic in British cattle. Scientists don't yet know how much BSE prion protein has to be consumed to contract CJD, or how much prion was contained in particular foodstuffs. The incubation period for the development of CJD is also unknown, but based on observations in people with classical CJD, it may be up to 40 years. In the light of these uncertainties, it is not really possible to make any predictions of the long-term impact of BSE on public health. New variant CJD has never been found in a country where BSE had not occurred.

human to human. There is no evidence that CJD can be spread in blood or blood products, but to be on the safe side, blood transfusion services have adopted regulations that require blood products derived from pooled blood to be produced from sources outside the United Kingdom.

In 1989 and 1996, legislation was passed to control animal feeding practices and to prevent high-risk cattle tissue from entering the food chain. This has resulted in a dramatic reduction in the number of new cases of BSE and has minimized the possibility of acquiring new variant CJD.

DEMENTIA
A persistent loss of memory and intellectual function that is severe enough to interfere with daily life.

We tend to associate dementia with elderly people and often see the condition as part of the natural aging process. In reality, dementia is a term used to describe symptoms that can be caused by a range of diseases and that can affect people of all ages.

What are the causes?
Damage to brain cells (neurons) or connecting fibers, or reduced amounts of chemical transmitters within the brain, can all lead to dementia.

- The cause of brain damage in Alzheimer's disease is believed to be the build-up of an abnormal protein in the neurons, which eventually kills these brain cells. Fewer neurons results in reduced levels of neurotransmitters, without which messages cannot pass along the nerves. In addition to old age, there appear to be additional risk factors for developing Alzheimer's disease, including family history, Down's syndrome, and serious head injury.
- Stroke causes at least 20 percent of all cases of dementia. Dementia can occur if a stroke affects the parts of the brain that perform intellectual functions such as speech, arithmetic, or memory. Dementia after stroke is more common in the elderly, in people with a lower level of education, and after more than one stroke.
- Parkinson's disease causes dementia in about 10 to 15 percent of people with the condition.
- Minor head injuries can cause bleeding; the resulting blood clot may compress the brain and mimic dementia.
- Toxic substances such as alcohol, prolonged exposure to some chemicals or heavy metals, or chemical imbalances caused by kidney dialysis or liver failure can all cause the symptoms of dementia.

- Frontal dementia and Picks disease are much less common. Symptoms often begin between the ages of 40 and 65 and are caused by the gradual destruction of neurons in the brain.
- Other rare causes of dementia include brain tumors, encephalitis, HIV infection, hydrocephalus, Creutzfeldt–Jakob disease, and Huntington's disease.

What are the symptoms?
The symptoms of dementia can be distressing both for the person with the disorder and for friends and family. The most frustrating symptom is undoubtedly memory loss and forgetfulness, which may become so severe that a person is unable to recognize loved ones, recall recent events, or remember familiar words. Learning new skills becomes practically impossible. As the disease progresses, a person may lose social skills and will appear to undergo a personality change, often becoming frustrated, restless, and agitated, and may wander aimlessly unless supervised.

How is it diagnosed?
Doctors will probably suspect a diagnosis of dementia following discussions with the family and observation of the person's behavior. Certain information will help doctors pinpoint the cause: The symptoms of some types of dementia, for example, develop at a younger age and have different rates of progression. There may also be a family history of a certain type of dementia.

Alzheimer's disease is the most common form of dementia; in the United States it affects about 10 percent of the population over 65 and half of those over 85.

In addition, doctors will usually perform tests on the brain such as magnetic resonance imaging (p. 108) or computed tomography scanning (p. 106) to look for evidence of previous strokes, bleeding, hydrocephalus, or brain tumors. Tests of higher brain function are frequently carried out to assess the stage of dementia, and blood may be tested to make sure that the symptoms are not caused by vitamin or hormone deficiencies, which are treatable.

What are the treatment options?
Some dementias resolve once the cause has been treated—for example, the successful removal of a brain tumor or blood clot. In most cases, though, damaged brain cells are impossible to repair, so treatment aims to slow down the disease rather than cure it, and to provide practical and emotional support. Alzheimer's can be treated with a group of drugs called anticholinesterases, which increase the

amount of a particular chemical transmitter—acetylcholine—in the brain. These drugs have been shown to improve memory and mental ability in people whose symptoms are not too severe. In all forms of dementia, it is possible to alleviate some of the distressing symptoms, such as depression or aggressive behavior, with medication.

DEPRESSION
One of a spectrum of mental illnesses called mood disorders. A common feature is a pervasive and persistent feeling of sadness, misery, or dejection.

Sadness and sorrow are emotions of normal experience that we all feel from time to time. The low mood of depression can be distinguished from these feelings by its greater intensity, duration, and pervasive quality. Mild depression may cause people to feel very sad and more tearful than usual. People who suffer moderate and severe depression experience overwhelming feelings of hopelessness, worthlessness, and failure, losing contact with their normal life and sense of well-being.

What is the cause?
Why do some people become depressed? Our knowledge about depression, although advancing, is incomplete. We do know, however, that a single cause is unlikely to be the answer. People probably have a degree of genetic vulnerability to depression that can be "activated" by additional life crises, such as a job loss, the break-up of a relationship, or sometimes a physical illness. There are also psychological vulnerabilities such as low self-esteem, or early childhood trauma, for example parental death or loss, that are more commonly associated with depression in later life. Some people seem to have such profound vulnerabilities that they do not need any added stress to become ill; developing depression seems to be a matter of when rather than if. An alternative theory suggests that depression is the result of an imbalance of particular chemicals in the brain called neurotransmitters.

What are the symptoms?
A doctor will ask about several symptoms associated with depression about before a diagnosis can be made; low mood is just one of them. It is important to establish that the person is different from his or her usual self, maybe in how he or she interacts with others or more usually in how he or she gets along in day-to-day life. This difference from

normal needs to be established for several weeks; it should coincide with several of the following symptoms:
- A low mood lasting for most of the day nearly every day
- Inability to enjoy the everyday things in life
- Losing weight and interest in food (or paradoxically, an increase in appetite, with weight gain).
- Difficulty sleeping, particularly waking up very early with a sense of dread
- Feeling sluggish, physically and mentally, nearly every day, or the opposite feeling of being irritable, agitated, restless, and unable to relax
- Feeling worthless, useless, and guilty
- Difficulty thinking clearly, focusing, or making decisions
- Experiencing recurring thoughts of death, wanting to die, or planning a suicide

When depression becomes severe, people can experience delusions, bizarre beliefs, or hallucinations.

How is it diagnosed?
To make a diagnosis of depression, a doctor has to take a psychiatric history and make an assessment of the person's mental state. This consists of a series of observations and questions to determine if someone has a depressed mood with some of the symptoms listed above and that these have lasted for some time. The questioning should also establish that several areas of the person's life have been disrupted.

What are the treatment options?
Drug therapy (p. 113) is just one area of treatment; others include psychological therapy and electroconvulsive therapy (p. 122). Antidepressants are thought to work by redressing the changes in brain chemicals—neurotransmitters—that commonly occur in depression. Psychological therapies can be effective alone or in combination with medication. Cognitive behavioral therapy is the most widely researched form of psychological treatment, which links feelings of depression to a person's negative thoughts about him- or herself and the world.

Electroconvulsive therapy has been used since the 1930s as a treatment for very severe depression.

What is the outlook?
Depression recurs for many people; some studies suggest more than half will experience another episode. The outlook is not good if bouts of depression are severe and frequent and a person does not completely recover in between episodes. Ongoing difficulties in relationships, social situations and unemployment reduce resilience to depression.

DIABETIC NERVE DAMAGE
Also known as diabetic neuropathy, this condition can result from uncontrolled diabetes mellitus.

Not everyone with diabetes mellitus develops what is known as diabetic neuropathy, in which the peripheral nerves become damaged. Good control of blood sugar levels significantly reduces the risk. Experts do not yet fully understand the cause of nerve damage; some think that it is probably caused by a combination of damage to the blood vessels and changes in the metabolism within cells as a result of abnormally high sugar levels. The doctor will probably already be on the lookout for any early signs of complications in a person with diabetes, including numbness and tingling in feet and hands, pain and weakness in the limbs, and constipation. An electrical test may be used to assess nerve function.

EPILEPSY
A disorder in which abnormal electrical discharges occur in the brain, resulting in a fit or seizure.

These days epilepsy, although extremely complex, is well understood and in most cases can be controlled with drugs. It is fairly common—in the United States it affects about 1 percent of the population, although 10 percent will have a seizure at some point in their lives. The seizures, which are the primary symptom of the disorder, vary immensely from individual to individual. In some people, there may be no more than a brief loss of concentration; in others, the seizure is more serious and affects the whole body.

For centuries, doctors were baffled by epilepsy, choosing to blame the seizures on hysteria, evil visitations, and mental illness.

What are the causes?
Experts are unable to find an obvious cause in more than 50 percent of people with epilepsy. There are, however, a few known causes of epilepsy: Sometimes the condition is inherited and occasionally it results from another disorder, such as a head injury, stroke, or brain tumor.

What are the symptoms?
Epileptic seizures are termed either "generalised," in which the abnormal electrical discharges affect the whole brain, or "partial," when they occur in only part of the brain. The most common form of generalized seizure is called tonic–clonic or *grand mal* and follows a particular pattern:

HELP YOUR DOCTOR TO HELP YOU

Being a good eyewitness
If you accompany a person with a reduced level of consciousness to the hospital, then any information you are able to provide is vital. Try to write down as many details as possible:

- *The person's age*
- *Any known medical problems, such as diabetes, stroke, or epilepsy*
- *Any known medication—if possible, take the drugs with you*

It is also very helpful if you can give extra descriptions, particularly if you were present when the person started to feel ill.

- *Was the onset gradual or sudden?*
- *What were the symptoms? For example, was the person pale, sweating, or having a seizure?*
- *What was the person doing at the time?*
- *Did the person sustain a blow to the head?*

All this information will provide crucial clues to help the doctors diagnose the problem.

- A sudden loss of consciousness; the person falls to the ground and becomes rigid
- Rhythmic jerking of the whole body lasting for up to a minute (rarely, tongue biting and incontinence occur)
- Continued unconsciousness for a few minutes to an hour

After a seizure, a person will wake slowly and appear confused as to his or her whereabouts. A headache, stiff limbs, and an overwhelming desire to sleep are common. Another form of generalized seizure is called an absence seizure, in which a person stops what he or she is doing and looks vague. Absence seizures are often first noticed when a child starts school, as he or she fails to keep up with classmates.

Partial seizures follow yet another pattern. The most common of these start in the frontal or temporal lobes of the brain. During a frontal seizure, the head and eyes deviate to one side, the arm on that side may jerk, and the person cannot speak. In a temporal seizure, the individual may notice an unpleasant smell or taste, or an intense emotion, for example fear or disgust.

How is it diagnosed?

Doctors cannot diagnose epilepsy on the basis of a single seizure, which may have another cause. When more than one seizure has occurred, however, the diagnosis is based mainly on an account of each episode. It is imperative that the doctor receives this account from an eyewitness, as the patient is often unable to give the full picture. Investigations of the brain often show normal results, although the doctor may still find some tests helpful in ruling out other conditions, such as a brain tumor. Measuring electrical activity in the brain (p. 111) with an electro-encephalogram may be helpful, and in some people the results show an abnormality. Brain imaging either with computed tomography scanning (p. 106) or magnetic resonance imaging (p. 108) may throw light on the cause of the epilepsy; scanning is done routinely on anyone over 30 to rule out a tumor.

What are the treatment options?

The treatment of choice for epilepsy is drug therapy (p. 118). Drugs need to be taken daily (often several times a day) for many years and often for life. In some people who have not experienced a seizure for a few years, it may be possible to withdraw the drugs. This is, however, always associated with the risk that seizures may recur. In a few individuals, neurosurgery (p. 122) to remove the abnormal area of the brain may be possible.

How can it be prevented or minimized?

The most important way to prevent seizures is by taking the drugs as directed by the doctor. Forgetting to take them, or deciding to miss a dose or stop the drugs altogether, can upset the brain's equilibrium and bring on a seizure. In addition, late nights, irregular eating, and flashing lights can all trigger a seizure, so it's wise to avoid them as far as possible.

HEAD INJURY

Damage to the head as a result of trauma with the potential risk of brain damage

In the United States, more than 230,000 people per year suffer head injuries requiring hospitalization. Most of these injuries are minor and have no lasting effects. Severe injury is rare, although head injury still accounts for one in four of all accidental deaths. More than half of all head injuries occur as a result of firearms use, whereas the remaining 50 percent are caused by other types of accidents (including traffic accidents), assaults, and sporting incidents. The most serious injuries are those in which the brain is damaged. A blow to the head can cause the brain to twist inside the skull; the side of the brain opposite the point of impact may be injured as the brain rocks back, hitting the other side of the skull. Bruising, bleeding, or even direct perforation with fragments of shattered skull or a heavy object can all occur in trauma.

What are the symptoms?

Head injuries are categorized into primary injury and secondary injury. The damage that occurs at the time of the accident is known as the primary injury and may include pain, swelling, bleeding, or laceration. Often, these injuries are minor and do not necessarily require medical attention. The crucial issue is whether a loss of consciousness occurred, however brief. In the hours following the initial head injury, further complications can occur—these are known as secondary injuries. The skull is a rigid box of fixed volume, so if bleeding or swelling occurs, the pressure will rise within. Left untreated, this raised pressure can cause coma and may be fatal. Watch out for the following symptoms; they can occur some time after the accident:

- Dizziness and nausea
- Memory loss and confusion
- Further loss of consciousness

Knowing when it's serious

If you witness a head injury, or if a friend or a family member has an accident, you may be undecided about what to do. It is advisable to seek urgent medical help (dial 911) if any of the following apply:

- *A loss of consciousness, however brief, has occurred.*

- *The wound on the head is bleeding profusely or appears deep.*

- *The person is bleeding from the ears or nose.*

- *Clear fluid is mixed with the blood.*

- *The person is confused, dizzy, nauseous, or appears to have memory loss.*

If you are in doubt or have any concerns, call your doctor anyway.

How is it diagnosed?

Usually, head injury will be obvious from a physical examination and medical history. If a person has lost consciousness, a skull X-ray (p. 104) will be taken to look for a fracture. The doctor will carry out a neurological examination, and if the patient's condition appears to be worsening, computed tomography scanning (p. 106) may be arranged to look for bleeding or swelling. If a person is confused or has a reduced level of consciousness, the Glasgow Coma Scale may be used to monitor progress.

What are the treatment options?

If the head injury did not cause loss of consciousness, a person is extremely unlikely to have a significant brain injury and may be discharged with no further investigation. If a brief loss of consciousness occurred, a period of observation is necessary, but in most cases recovery is rapid and further treatment is not necessary. Severely injured patients will be monitored and treated in an intensive care unit and will probably be artificially ventilated, which can help reduce the pressure inside the brain. If a blood clot is seen on CT scanning, emergency surgery (p. 122) may be required to remove the clot.

What is the outcome?

Most people with head injuries recover fully and have no further problems. Severe injuries, however, may have long-term consequences that can be devastating. Memory and concentration difficulties, speech and motor difficulties, and emotional instability can follow a severe injury.

HYDROCEPHALUS

A build-up of fluid in the ventricles of the brain causes an increase in the pressure within the skull.

In the center of the brain are fluid-filled spaces called ventricles, which produce cerebrospinal fluid (CSF). This vital fluid circulates around the brain and spinal cord, protecting and nourishing the cells, and is eventually absorbed into the bloodstream. If there is an abnormal increase in the amount of CSF, the ventricles become enlarged—a condition known as hydrocephalus.

What are the causes?

Hydrocephalus is caused in one of two ways: Either a blockage occurs in the drainage system so that CSF is unable to drain away and builds up inside the ventricles, or too much CSF is produced. Usually, hydrocephalus is present at birth and develops because of an abnormal narrowing of one of the channels through which CSF normally flows. In some babies, hydrocephalus occurs in association with another condition such as spina bifida. On rare occasions, hydrocephalus develops as a consequence of meningitis, a brain tumor, or a head injury.

What are the symptoms?

The symptoms of hydrocephalus differ depending on the age of the affected person. A baby or young child with hydrocephalus may have a distinctive physical appearance as the bones of the skull are not fused and the increased pressure inside the brain (from the extra CSF) can result in abnormal head enlargement. In older children or adults, the increase in pressure may cause nausea, vomiting, and headache. Furthermore, older children usually have difficulty walking and may be slow to develop intellectually.

How is it diagnosed?

If the ventricles are widened or the baby's head is beginning to enlarge, the condition can often be diagnosed before birth with a routine scan, or after delivery. In all cases of suspected hydrocephalus, doctors will scan the brain—either with computed tomography scanning (p. 106) or, in babies, ultrasound scanning (p. 110)—to see whether there is an obvious cause for the condition.

What are the treatment options?

If the cause can be treated—for example, a tumor can be removed—then the hydrocephalus may be cured. In some people, the build-up of pressure reaches a certain point and then does not progress any further, so treatment may not be necessary. Otherwise, doctors will probably decide to insert a shunt into the brain to drain away the excess CSF. A shunt is a long piece of tubing that passes down through the body from the ventricle in the brain into the heart, the abdomen, or a lung cavity, where the excess CSF is harmlessly absorbed.

What is the outlook?

The outlook really depends on the severity of the condition, the timeliness of the treatment, and whether it is successful. Without treatment, or sometimes even despite it, the raised pressure in the brain has a damaging effect on the tissue itself and can lead to physical disabilities and learning difficulties. Some people, however, live normal lives.

MENINGITIS

Inflammation of the meninges (membranes around the brain) usually caused by a viral or a bacterial infection.

Meningitis is one of the most feared diseases that affects children and adults alike. Viral meningitis mainly affects young adults and is the more common but usually less severe form. Bacterial meningitis develops predominantly in children and, although rare, can be life threatening. Both viruses and bacteria can travel in the bloodstream from other parts of the body or can be transmitted to the brain from nearby structures, such as the sinuses, throat, or ears.

What are the symptoms?

Thanks to the media and public health campaigns, many people are aware of the classic symptoms of meningitis:
• Raised temperature
• Neck stiffness and dislike of bright lights
• Headache and drowsiness
These symptoms often come on rapidly, but in some cases of meningitis, for example those caused by a virus, or tubercular meningitis, the onset is more gradual, and symptoms may simply consist of mild aches and pains and a slight temperature. In very young children, the following symptoms may develop:
• A reluctance to eat
• Vomiting
• Floppiness
• Fits or seizures

Should everyone be immunized against meningitis?

TALKING POINT

Vaccines now exist that can protect against most strains of bacterial meningitis. None protect against group B, one of the most common strains in the United States, however. The vaccines are not effective in children under 18 months, nor are they routinely recommended in the United States. Recently, however, the Centers for Disease Control has advised that college freshmen, who are at a moderately increased risk for the disease, receive the meningococcal vaccine. Anyone planning to travel outside the country, in particular to Africa and Asia, should consult a doctor well in advance of the trip to discuss which meningitis vaccines are recommended.

One type of bacterial meningitis, meningococcal meningitis, causes a rash of reddish-purple spots that don't fade when pressed with the side of a glass—this is known as a purpuric rash and indicates that the condition is serious.

How is it diagnosed?

A physical examination (p. 100) may enable the doctor to make a diagnosis of meningitis right away, especially if there is a purpuric rash. If this is the case, hospital admission should be arranged as soon as possible. Once in a hospital, the diagnosis is usually confirmed by the examination of a sample of cerebrospinal fluid obtained through a spinal tap (p. 103). If there is a bacterial infection, it will show up in the spinal fluid and will also grow in the laboratory in a sample of blood. Viruses are much harder to detect. Scanning the brain using computed tomography (p. 106) or magnetic resonance imaging (p. 108) may be useful to exclude other diagnoses such as stroke or abscess.

What are the treatment options?

As soon as meningitis is suspected, the doctor will arrange admission to hospital for assessment, tests, and treatment. There is no treatment for viral meningitis—antibiotics are not effective against viruses—and the symptoms usually resolve themselves spontaneously. In these cases, if a person is well enough, he or she may be discharged, to be followed up by medical staff on a regular basis.

Bacterial meningitis, however, should be treated as soon as possible with antibiotics, which are given as an injection into the bloodstream so they can start working immediately— even before the test results are confirmed. A person with bacterial meningitis is often very unwell and may need to be looked after in an intensive care unit. If a person has seizures, anticonvulsant drugs and steroids may be prescribed to reduce brain swelling.

What is the outcome?

Even though almost all of us are aware of the symptoms of bacterial meningitis, about 15 percent of all people who contract the condition do not survive. The risk is heightened if diagnosis and treatment are delayed, if a person already has another illness such as diabetes, or if the immune system is faulty. The elderly and the very young often take longer to recover than other age groups.

MIGRAINE

A severe headache, which usually comes on gradually over a period of up to several hours and can last from three hours to three days.

Migraine is a severe type of headache that can be extremely debilitating. Most migraines occur infrequently, and symptoms can usually be controlled with drugs and/or lifestyle changes.

What are the causes?

Migraines are thought to be related to abnormal behavior in certain blood vessels in the brain, but experts are unsure about the exact cause. Just before symptoms start, the small arteries in the brain become narrowed, so that blood flow is reduced. It appears that the headache itself begins when these same arteries suddenly widen. The reason for this excessive activity is unclear but there do appear to be certain triggers. Menstruation, stress, sleep deprivation, sexual intercourse, fever, and caffeine withdrawal may all initiate a migraine attack in some people. A genetic factor may be involved, because the condition runs in families.

Chocolate, red wine, and cheese are all thought to trigger migraines in some people.

What are the symptoms?

Many people receive some kind of warning that a migraine is imminent—this is sometimes known as an "aura" or a "prodrome." During this time, a person may feel nauseous, yawn excessively, crave sweet foods, or see flashing lights, stars, or zigzag lines; sometimes, half the field of vision will disappear. These symptoms last for about 15 to 30 minutes and then the migraine starts. The pain is often felt on only one side of the head and is usually so severe that the person just wants to lie down in a dark room and sleep.

How is it diagnosed?

Migraine is usually diagnosed after the doctor has taken a history of the symptoms. Rarely, a brain scan may be done, but only if the doctor suspects a more serious reason for the headache, such as a tumor.

What are the treatment options?

Often, the onset of migraine can be frightening, and people need to be reassured that there is nothing worse wrong with them. The symptoms can usually be relieved with medication, and often a simple pain-relieving drug such as paracetamol will do the trick. There are two types of specific drugs for

HAVING A MIGRAINE

My first migraine was frightening.... I actually thought I was going blind. Half of my vision suddenly went—the kind of blindness you get when someone has taken a photograph of you with a flash camera.

I don't know how long it lasted but then this throbbing pain on one side of my head started. I felt sick and dizzy but my sight had come back. It was all I could do to call the doctor and struggle upstairs to bed. I honestly believed that I was having a stroke.

Eventually, when my doctor diagnosed migraine I felt a mixture of relief and anxiety. She said that it all had to do with the blood flow in my brain. In migraine, blood vessels suddenly become narrowed and restrict blood flow to the eye—hence the problems with my vision—and the brain. This constriction is followed by the vessels widening, which stimulates nearby pain receptors. Once blood flow returns to normal, the pain subsides.

migraine (p. 115) available—those that treat the symptoms and those that prevent a migraine from occurring. The doctor will prescribe medication according to the frequency of the migraines and the severity of the symptoms.

Can it be prevented or minimized?

A person should try to identify whether there are any common triggers preceding the migraine attacks, then avoid the trigger substance or behavior.

MOTOR NEURON DISEASE

A rare, progressive, slow-developing disease that affects the nerves in the brain and spinal cord—motor neurons—that control movement.

The debilitating symptoms of motor neuron disease (MND) usually first appear in people over the age of 40. Over the course of the disease, the muscles involved in movement gradually waste away. In most cases, the cause is unknown, but experts believe that there may be a genetic element to MND—in 5 to 10 percent of people affected, other members of the family also have the disease.

What are the symptoms?

Usually, MND starts slowly; at first, an affected person may not realize anything is wrong. Gradually he or she may start to stumble or may notice a weak grip, muscle stiffness, and difficulty climbing stairs. Sometimes, the muscles that control speech and swallowing are affected. As the disease progresses, muscle weakness becomes worse, and in the later stages, speech and swallowing may become impossible. Although the condition results in very severe physical disability, a person's senses and intelligence remain unaffected, as does bladder and bowel function.

How is it diagnosed?

Doctors may not diagnose MND right away because the symptoms are so insidious. When symptoms first develop, they tend to be fairly general and could indicate any number of disorders. As a result, a person may have to undergo a variety of tests before the correct diagnosis is made; there is no specific test for MND. Magnetic resonance imaging (p. 108) may be done to check for a disease of the spinal cord, and a spinal tap (p. 103) will confirm whether there is any inflammation in the spinal fluid. A test known as electromyelography can show if nerves supplying the muscles are damaged.

What are the treatment options?

Currently there is no treatment available either to slow down the progression of MND or to cure it. Treatment focuses on the relief of symptoms, and a variety of professionals will meet with the family to plan each individual's care. Physical therapy and occupational therapy are vital to keep the limbs as supple as possible and to avoid painful spasms and cramps. If swallowing becomes impossible, doctors usually insert a small tube directly into the stomach through which liquid food can be given. The provision of a communication aid, with a keyboard and screen, can often help a person who becomes unable to speak. In some people, the disease affects the muscles that control breathing and it may eventually be necessary to use a breathing machine—a ventilator—for periods of time.

What is the outlook?

Because of the lack of effective treatment and the progressive nature of the disease, the outlook for MND sufferers is not good. Some people live for 10 years or more, but in others, particularly those whose condition deteriorated rapidly in the first months after diagnosis, the condition may be fatal within 3 years.

MULTIPLE SCLEROSIS
A condition that damages the nerves of the brain and spinal cord, causing varying degrees of disability.

Many of the nerves in the central nervous system are surrounded by protective sheaths made from a fatty substance called myelin, which speeds transmission of messages along the nerves. For reasons that are yet unclear, the myelin sheaths become damaged in people with multiple sclerosis (MS), which interferes with message transmission. How the disease manifests itself varies enormously— a person may have only a single episode and then never experience another one. Other sufferers have frequent attacks with recovery in between, known as relapsing remitting MS. If symptoms continue to worsen with no recovery, the condition is termed chronic progressive MS.

What are the causes?

Experts continue to research the cause, but currently it remains a mystery. Some theories suggest that MS may be an autoimmune disorder, or that it is triggered by a virus or environmental factors. Interestingly, the condition is much more common in certain areas: Temperate regions, such as northern Europe, have a much higher incidence of MS than the tropics, where the condition is rare. Genetic factors are important—the risk of developing MS is higher if a person has a close relative with the condition.

What are the symptoms?

The first symptoms of MS usually develop in young people over the age of 20 and depend largely on which nerves are damaged. There is no such thing as a typical attack— symptoms may last for days or weeks and then disappear for months or years. The optic nerve, which relays visual information from the eye to the brain, is commonly affected, so that vision is blurred and the eye may be painful. If the nerve is severely damaged, sight may be lost completely. Damaged nerves elsewhere in the brain and spinal cord can result in weakness, numbness, and tingling anywhere in the body. People with MS may be unsteady on their feet and suffer from dizziness. If the nerves supplying the bladder are involved, there may be problems with passing urine—a desperate urge to go to the toilet far more often than usual and sometimes even incontinence. Men may find that they are unable to achieve an erection. Many people with MS suffer frequent fatigue, and as the disease progresses, concentration, and memory problems (especially short-term memory) and depression are common.

Should marijuana be prescribed for MS sufferers?

The treatments available to treat MS are still far from effective: Even the newest drugs offer only small increases in quality of life for a few people. It is understandable then that sufferers are willing to try anything that may help. Some MS sufferers have confirmed that marijuana usage relieves their painful muscle spasms and tremors. Despite this, there have been few proper scientific trials, although research (mostly in Britain) is ongoing. Research into the effects of cannabis, the active ingredient in marijuana, is difficult because using the substance is illegal in the United States. Prohibition hurts drug trials in two ways: People with MS who use marijuana are reluctant to admit it, and proper trials of its effects on patients who may benefit are almost impossible to conduct. Trials are now underway, but it will be some time before we have a scientific answer to the question, does marijuana really help MS sufferers?

How is it diagnosed?

Doctors do not usually make the diagnosis of MS until there have been two or more episodes, separated by at least a few weeks and involving different parts of the central nervous system. Magnetic resonance imaging (p. 108) usually shows up abnormal areas in the brain, which may suggest MS. It is also possible to measure how messages pass along nerves using tests called visual evoked responses.

What are the treatment options?

There is currently no cure for MS, and there appears to be little that can be done to halt the progress of the condition. A particularly severe attack of MS may be treated with steroid drugs. Over the past few years, a new drug called interferon-beta has reduced the number of attacks and the level of disability in certain circumstances. It is still too early to say if the drug will be of long-term benefit. Physical therapy and occupational therapy play vital roles in helping an individual remain mobile and independent.

What is the outlook?

MS appears to be more severe in men, in people who develop it later in life, and in those who have several attacks in quick succession early on in the illness. Many people with relapsing MS lead normal lives during the periods of remission; those with chronic progressive MS, however, often become increasingly disabled.

MYELITIS

Weakness and numbness in the limbs and trunk resulting from an inflamed spinal cord.

If the delicate spinal cord, normally well protected by the backbone, becomes inflamed, any spinal nerves that branch from the inflamed area are also affected and cause symptoms in the areas of the body that they supply. Inflammation of the spinal cord (also known as myelitis) can be a serious condition that can cause lasting disability.

What are the causes?

Myelitis has many possible causes, which can be broadly classified into infectious and noninfectious. Infectious agents include viruses, such as those that cause poliomyelitis and shingles, and the human immunodeficiency virus (HIV); bacteria, for example those that cause syphilis and tuberculosis; and parasites and fungi. Other causative conditions include multiple sclerosis and certain vaccinations, such as a certain type of rabies vaccine.

What are the symptoms?

Weakness in both legs is often the first indication that something is wrong—the arms are not usually affected. If the condition is particularly severe, a person may lose bladder control or be left with long-term stiffness in the limbs. The symptoms can appear and progress over a matter of days or over a few weeks.

How is it diagnosed?

Following a physical examination (p. 100) to establish where the spinal cord is affected, the doctor may request magnetic resonance imaging (p. 108) of the back or neck. In addition, a person with myelitis will probably have blood tests (p. 101) and a spinal tap (p. 103), both of which can indicate infection and inflammation.

What are the treatment options?

The treatment depends on the cause of the inflammation, and there are many. If the culprit is an infection, it can sometimes be treated with antimicrobial drugs. Myelitis with a noninfectious cause, particularly an acute attack of multiple sclerosis, can be treated effectively with steroids.

PARKINSON'S DISEASE

A progressive nervous system disorder with very distinctive symptoms—a combination of tremor, stiffness, and slow movement.

People over the age of 50 are the group most affected by Parkinson's disease. The condition is not uncommon—it affects about 20 people in every 100,000 per year. Much research is currently being done on Parkinson's disease as experts try to find both a cure for the disease and a way of reducing the often distressing physical symptoms.

What is the cause?

The part of the brain called the basal ganglia, which is responsible for producing smooth muscle movements, degenerates in someone with Parkinson's disease. A chemical called dopamine, normally produced by cells in the basal ganglia, coordinates movement with the help of another chemical known as acetylcholine; these two neurotransmitters have opposing but finely balanced actions. Dopamine is in short supply in someone with Parkinson's disease, so there is a chemical imbalance in the brain and the effect of acetylcholine predominates.

What are the symptoms?

During the early stages of Parkinson's disease, the symptoms usually affect one side of the body only. A tremor in the hand, slowness of movement, and stiff limbs may be the first signs of the disease, and even turning over in bed can be a problem. As the condition progresses, both sides of the body become affected and a person may start to have difficulty articulating words. Often, the face loses its expression and becomes almost mask-like. Eventually, the reflexes that help us to maintain an upright posture on an uneven surface are lost, resulting in frequent falls.

Symptoms similar to those of Parkinson's disease can arise as a side effect of certain drugs, following repeated head injuries, or after a case of viral encephalitis; in these cases, the condition is known as Parkinsonism.

How is it diagnosed?

Often the doctor will immediately be able to identify the classic signs of Parkinson's disease—tremor, stiffness, and slow movements. A careful history of other illnesses and details of any drugs will be taken to exclude causes of Parkinsonism. Computed tomography scanning (p. 106) or magnetic resonance imaging (p. 108) may show some brain shrinkage, but scans are usually normal.

What are the treatment options?

Currently the primary therapy is drugs (p. 119), although research is underway to find alternative solutions. Some drugs work only for a limited period and so treatment is generally not started until symptoms begin to affect a person's lifestyle. Drug treatment aims to restore the balance of dopamine and acetylcholine in the brain.

Surgery is sometimes an option for people with severe Parkinson's disease that has not responded very well to drug treatment. It is possible to remove the overactive parts of the basal ganglia or to stimulate the underactive parts.

Recently, some people with Parkinson's disease have been given an implant, similar to a heart pacemaker, which delivers electrical impulses to the brain; this helps to control tremors and stiffness.

What is the outcome?

Many people with Parkinson's disease are able to lead full and active lives with the help of drug therapy. In the long term, however, the symptoms become more difficult to control and this may mean that a sufferer will need more and more help in getting around and performing basic tasks. The condition has inspired a great deal of medical research and hopefully new, more effective treatments will be available in the not too distant future.

PHENYLKETONURIA

A very rare, inherited chemical imbalance in the brain that can cause brain damage.

All babies in the United States are routinely tested for phenylketonuria a few days after birth. As a result, the condition is usually detected early in life and can be treated quickly before symptoms develop. A baby with phenylketonuria is missing an enzyme that breaks down a substance called phenylalanine, which is found in protein-rich food. At high levels, phenylalanine is converted into chemicals that can damage brain tissue.

If undetected at birth, the condition usually begins to show symptoms during the first year of life, and the diagnosis is confirmed with a blood test. Treatment involves restricting phenylalanine in the diet; this usually continues for life. If the special diet is started early after diagnosis, children with phenylketonuria develop normally. Children whose treatment is delayed, however, may have learning difficulties and need special care.

SCHIZOPHRENIA
A serious mental illness in which there is a loss of sense of reality and an inability to function socially.

Our knowledge about schizophrenia is advancing, but it is far from complete. Schizophrenia affects about 1 to 1.5 percent of the population in the United States, and the genetic contribution to the illness is probably about 50 percent. However, we have not yet identified the gene responsible. As with other mental illnesses, this genetic contribution forms a vulnerability, and other events are required before a person develops the syndrome. Other theories include a complicated birth and a viral infection during early pregnancy. The actual onset of the illness is frequently preceded by a stressful event; stress acts as a precipitant and is also associated with relapses of the illness over time.

What are the symptoms?
The symptoms of schizophrenia are divided into two categories: positive symptoms and negative symptoms.
- **Positive symptoms** These are the more bizarre or abnormal experiences and include hallucinations, including hearing voices. These experiences are very real and frequently terrifying. Delusions are false and often unusual beliefs that the schizophrenic holds to be absolutely true; these are frequently persecutory in nature. Other "positive symptoms" include a feeling of being controlled by external forces or having thoughts inserted or taken out of the person's mind.
- **Negative symptoms** These include a reduced interest in surroundings and an inability or decreased ability to experience pleasure or desire. The person appears withdrawn and emotionally blank and cannot be engaged in lengthy or detailed conversation. Some of the longer term symptoms in severe schizophrenia are the disruption of normal relationships and the limited ability to work or to lead an independent life.

How is it diagnosed?
Diagnosing a first episode of schizophrenia can sometimes be difficult because other illness, such as severe depression, may have similar symptoms. There is no specific test for schizophrenia, and the doctor will make a diagnosis only after careful questioning and observation of the person. Family members and friends can also contribute to the overall picture by describing any changes in a person's personality or behavior. Often the condition will not be confirmed until one or more episodes have occurred.

What are the treatment options?
There are now a variety of treatments available for schizophrenia. Antipsychotic drugs (p. 119) are traditionally useful in treating only positive symptoms. Nowadays, newer forms of medication—known as "atypical antipsychotics"—can improve negative symptoms.

Rehabilitation is an important part of treatment because the illness can affect the person's ability to lead a normal life. Support is provided by members of the community mental health team, who help the person with daily activities, work, social contacts, living arrangements, and claiming insurance benefits. Sheltered work placements and residential care are also available for people with severe illness. Psychotherapy can help with current symptoms and decrease the chance of relapse in the future. Newer forms of cognitive therapy addressing the positive symptoms of the illness have been developed and have had promising results.

Contrary to popular belief, very few people with schizophrenia are dangerous—they are far more at risk of harming themselves than others. Sometimes a person will refuse much needed treatment because of the stigma attached to the illness. In such cases it may be necessary to detain patients in hospital against their will. (Most states in this country have laws to permit some form of involuntary commitment, but this remains a controversial issue.)

What is the outlook?
Schizophrenia is an illness with a broad spectrum of severity and duration. After the first episode, about 25 percent of people will make a good recovery, about 60 percent will have episodes of acute illness with good periods in between, and a smaller percentage (about 15 percent) develop a severe and debilitating illness.

SHINGLES
An infectious, painful rash of watery blisters caused by a virus that develops along a nerve pathway.

Shingles is uncommon in young, healthy people and usually only affects the elderly or those whose immune systems are not functioning as well as they should. When it does occur, shingles is a painful and distressing condition. A shingles rash has a characteristic appearance because it affects a nerve pathway and so usually develops in a band-like pattern on one side of the body, around the ribcage and abdomen, but can develop on the face and eyes. Shingles is caused by the virus herpes zoster, which also causes chicken pox. After an episode of chicken pox, the virus stays in the body but lies dormant. In some people, however, the virus can be reactivated and causes shingles. People with shingles should avoid contact with vulnerable people; the blisters are infectious and can result in chicken pox in a person not already immune

What are the symptoms?
The symptoms of shingles occur in three stages. First, you may feel a pricking, tingling sensation or a sharp pain in the affected area. Soon afterward, small watery blisters erupt on the skin. A few days later, the blisters dry out and scab over—don't be tempted to pull these off; this can lead to scarring. After the scabs have disappeared, there is usually no visible scarring, although the skin may remain slightly darker in the affected area.

How is it diagnosed?
The doctor will usually be able to diagnose shingles once the rash has developed. Prior to that, it is possible to mistake the pain, especially if it is severe, for a heart attack. If there is some doubt, a sample of tissue from the shingles blisters can be examined under a microscope.

What are the treatment options?
The sooner treatment is started, the less severe and long-lasting the attack. The doctor will probably prescribe an antiviral drug (usually aciclovir) in tablet form; if the eye is affected, aciclovir also comes as ointment or eye drops.

Shingles usually clears up within two to six weeks. The pain of shingles, however, may persist for some months after the rash has healed, a condition known as postherpetic neuralgia. An episode of shingles does not provide immunity, so in some people the condition recurs.

SLEEP DISORDERS
Persistent disturbances of sleeping patterns, such as sleeping too little or too much, sudden sleep attacks, night terrors, and jet lag.

Sleep disturbances that persist are a cause of great distress and may take several forms.
- **Insomnia** Sleeping too little can have a variety of physical or psychological causes, for example a depressive or anxiety disorder, an alcohol problem, certain drugs (particularly caffeine), medical conditions, or disruptions to normal daily routines. When no underlying cause seems apparent, psychological reasons such as stress and anger may be responsible.
- **Narcolepsy** An irresistible urge to sleep is a rare disorder and is thought to be genetically determined.
- **Parasomnias** Sleep walking and night terrors are common in childhood but persist in only 1 to 2 percent of the adult population. Children in the same families tend to be affected, suggesting a genetic vulnerability. In adults, parasomnias are frequently triggered by stress or even certain drugs or alcohol.

What are the symptoms?
The main symptom of insomnia is difficulty achieving or maintaining sleep; this is frequently accompanied by daytime sleepiness, which disrupts normal functioning. Narcolepsy's characteristic symptom is the irresistible onset of sleep at inappropriate times, even when the person is absorbed in a task. It can be accompanied by sudden attacks of muscular weakness (cataplexy), the experience of being suddenly unable to move just on the point of sleeping or waking (sleep paralysis), and hallucinations that occur as the person is waking or falling asleep. Night terrors are particularly disturbing for bed partners because sufferers may scream suddenly and panic as if in real danger. Most people have little or no memory of the events the next day.

How is it diagnosed?
To assess a sleep disorder, a doctor will often request that the person's partner is present to add relevant information. Also, a sleep diary in which a person notes sleep patterns and specific symptoms can be useful.

The person may be referred to a sleep specialist for further tests because psychological questionnaires uncover information about current problems and personality traits. Other more extensive tests such as measurement of brainwave patterns and muscle and eye movements during sleep (polysomnography) at home or in hospital can be useful.

We spend about one-third of our lives asleep. One of the most common reasons for visiting the doctor is a sleep problem.

What are the treatment options?
Since the causes of insomnia are multiple, the first line of treatment is to identify and treat the relevant ones. The next aim is to develop a regular sleep routine:
- Going to bed and getting up at the same time each day
- Resisting daytime naps
- Avoiding stimulants, such as caffeine, and alcohol

- Not exercising before bedtime
- Keeping the bedroom at a constant cool temperature
- Eating regular meals

If sleep refuses to come, it may help to get up and read or make a milky drink until sleepiness returns. Sedatives are recommended only as a short-term measure (two weeks maximum, because of their addictive qualities), when sleeplessness has come about because of a crisis, such as a bereavement.

There are no curative treatments for narcolepsy, so treatment aims to reduce the impact of the symptoms on quality of life. Behavioral measures such as taking small naps are helpful in capitalizing on the alert state following the attacks. Stimulants can help to reduce daytime sleepiness or improve muscle tone. Support groups are important.

Parasomnias are difficult to treat, and sleep hygiene is important. Low-dose Valium-like drugs, or some of the newer antidepressants, have been useful for some patients but have made matters worse in others.

SPINA BIFIDA
A condition caused by abnormal fetal development of the vertebrae and spinal cord.

A baby's spinal cord and its coverings develop from the neural tube during the first few weeks of pregnancy. Spina bifida occurs if there is a defect in the tube and the backbone develops abnormally. If the abnormality is confined to the bones themselves, it is called spina bifida occulta. If the spinal cord or nerve roots are involved, it is called spina bifida cystica.

What are the causes?
The number of people affected by spina bifida in the United States has decreased dramatically over recent decades, probably because of advances in prenatal care and health education. Although doctors are unclear as to the exact cause of spina bifida, there do appear to be several factors that increase the risk of having a baby with the condition. A couple who already has a child with spina bifida has a 2 to 4 percent risk in subsequent pregnancies. It also appears that older women have a higher risk of having an affected child.

What are the symptoms?
Babies with spina bifida occulta develop normally, and often the only outward sign may be a mole or a hairy patch at the base of the spine. If the spinal cord and nerve roots are involved, however, an affected baby may have

neurological problems, particularly if the abnormality is high up on the spine. In these instances, the symptoms may be severe and often include the following:
- Leg weakness and deformities
- Numbness affecting the legs and bottom
- Incontinence

The majority of children with spina bifida cystica also have an excessive amount of fluid around the brain, a condition known as hydrocephalus (p. 143).

How is it diagnosed?
Often, doctors are able to confirm during pregnancy that a baby has spina bifida by using a combination of blood tests and ultrasound scans. If the diagnosis is not made during the pregnancy, then the condition may be obvious when the baby is born. X-rays (p. 104) and magnetic resonance imaging (p. 108) of the spine will confirm the diagnosis.

What are the treatment options?
Babies with spina bifida occulta do not often need treatment. Usually, doctors operate on babies with spina bifida cystica to close the spinal defect within the first few days of life. It is important to carry out the surgery as soon as possible to prevent infection from entering the spinal cord and causing meningitis. Later in life, children often need further operations to correct limb deformities and bypass the bladder. A baby who also has hydrocephalus may need a shunt inserted to drain excess fluid away from the brain.

How can it be prevented or minimized?
A woman who is planning a pregnancy should ideally take a folic acid supplement for three months before she conceives and for the first three months of pregnancy; this significantly reduces the risk of spina bifida.

SPINAL INJURY AND PARALYSIS
Varying degrees of loss of sensation in the body following trauma to the spinal column.

The most common causes of spinal injuries are traffic accidents, falls, and sporting injuries—soccer, horseback riding and diving into shallow water being among the higher risk pursuits. An injury occurs when the bones and ligaments of the spinal column are damaged, allowing the spinal cord to be severely twisted or stretched. As a result, the nerves passing down the spine are disrupted and messages cannot travel beyond the level of the injury.

What are the symptoms?

A person with spinal damage often has severe injuries to other parts of the body, particularly the head. Symptoms of spinal injury may include

- Unconsciousness
- Visible injury to the back or an abnormal lying position
- Pain at the site of the injury
- Altered sensation in the lower part of the body
- Inability to move

How is it diagnosed?

The doctor can usually make a fairly accurate diagnosis of spinal injury following a physical examination (p. 100). X-rays (p. 104), computed tomography scanning (p. 106), and magnetic resonance imaging (p. 108) will confirm the exact location of the injury and the extent of the damage to the spine.

What are the treatment options?

The treatment depends on the severity of the injury. Fractures can be stabilized with traction, but other injuries are more long term. Nerve tissue cannot regenerate once it has been damaged, so treatment centers on rehabilitation. Many people with spinal injuries require hospital admission that, in severe cases, may last for months or even years. A multidisciplinary team carries out an individualized rehabilitation program to help a person regain independence. This program involves intensive physical therapy and occupational therapy to regain as much function as possible and to adapt to a new life.

What is the outlook?

Where the injury occurs is important in assessing the outlook. The higher up the spine the injury, the more severe the paralysis. For example, a severe injury at neck level would prevent messages from traveling down the length of the spinal cord, causing complete paralysis (quadraplegia). An injury affecting the nerves supplying the respiratory muscles may be fatal. An injury lower down the spine would spare the arms but would paralyze both legs (paraplegia), whose nerves emerge from the lumbar segments of the spinal cord. Much hope recently has focused on drug treatments that might allow the nerves to regrow back down the damaged spinal cord, but this is not yet an option.

In the United States each year, about 7,600 to 11,000 people receive an injury to the spinal cord that often results in devastating paralysis and loss of sensation.

STROKE

A sudden disturbance in the function of the brain because of a blockage in the blood supply or a ruptured blood vessel. Symptoms lasting fewer than 24 hours are called transient ischemic attacks.

Whether a stroke results from a blocked blood vessel or from internal bleeding in the brain, the results are similar: damage to the surrounding brain tissue, with potentially long-term and disabling consequences. Disruption of the brain's blood supply can occur for the following reasons.

- **Hardening of the arteries** Known as atherosclerosis, this is the most common cause of stroke. In this condition, arteries becomes clogged up and narrowed by fatty deposits called plaque so that blood is unable to flow easily through the vessel. A fragment of plaque can become dislodged and travel round the brain in the bloodstream until it blocks a narrower artery. Alternatively, a plaque in an artery in the brain can gradually increase in size until it completely blocks the vessel. The carotid artery, which supplies the majority of blood to the brain, is a common site of atherosclerosis. Atherosclerosis develops in all of us as we age, but the process happens faster in smokers and in people with high blood pressure or diabetes.
- **Heart disease** If one of the chambers of the heart is faulty and does not contract as it should, for example after a heart attack, a clot can form on the lining of the chamber. If the clot is dislodged, it can be carried to the brain in the bloodstream, where it can block a small artery. Clots may also form in conditions in which the heartbeat is irregular.
- **Abnormal blood vessels** A weakened or malformed blood vessel deep in the brain tissue can rupture and cause a stroke. Sometimes, persistently high blood pressure can eventually lead to bleeding within the brain.

What are the symptoms?

Stroke happens suddenly with little or no warning, and symptoms are often frightening. How each individual is affected depends on which area of the brain has been damaged. For example, a stroke in the left side of the brain can lead to sudden weakness and loss of feeling in the right side of the body and speech and swallowing difficulties. If the stroke occurs in the back of the brain, a person may have problems with balance. Level of consciousness can be affected by all kinds of stroke. If a sudden bleed occurs within brain tissue, a person may develop a severe headache and rapidly become unconscious.

How is it diagnosed?

The doctor will usually be able to tell whether a person has had a stroke by the symptoms and from a physical examination (p. 100). Imaging the brain using techniques such as computed tomography scanning (p. 106) or magnetic resonance imaging (p. 108) can help to confirm the diagnosis and locate the area of damage.

What are the treatment options?

Most people who have suffered a stroke are admitted to the hospital very quickly. The treatment will then depend on the cause of the stroke.

- If the stroke is caused by a clot, drugs (p. 120) may be given to thin the blood and prevent further clots from developing. Sometimes a drug is used to dissolve an existing clot. If the person suffering the stroke has an irregular heartbeat, heart-regulating drugs will probably be prescribed. Ultrasound scanning (p. 110) of the carotid arteries may be done—If narrowing of the vessels is confirmed, then surgery to remove the narrowed area may be possible. An alternative to surgery is angioplasty, during which a catheter is inserted into an artery in the groin and then threaded up the vessel until it reaches the narrowed part of the carotid artery. Once in place, a tiny balloon at the catheter's tip is inflated to stretch the area.

Twenty percent of the blood that is pumped out from the heart goes straight to the brain.

- If the stroke is due to bleeding, a neurosurgeon may decide to operate to remove the resulting clot, particularly if it is large and is pressing on vital structures. A contrast X-ray (p. 104), called an angiogram, is of great value in assessing which blood vessels in the brain are damaged. Angiography is not normally done until about six weeks after the stroke, except in cases of subarachnoid hemorrhage, when it is done as soon as possible. If any abnormalities show up on the angiogram, surgery or specialist treatment using X-ray techniques can be used to remove the abnormality and prevent further bleeds.

Treatment for stroke victims is most effective if it is carried out by what is known as a multi-disciplinary team, including nurses, physical therapists, occupational therapists, speech therapists, dietitians, and doctors experienced in the management of stroke, who work together in a coordinated fashion. The rate and extent of recovery varies immensely from person to person depending on the extent of damage to the brain and the severity of any resulting disability.

HAVING A STROKE

I am 57 years old, and was at work when I first noticed an odd numb sensation down my left arm. Very quickly it spread to the whole of my left side—I couldn't move!

I tried to get up from my chair to get a glass of water, but my legs wouldn't work, and I fell onto the floor. I tried to shout out to my colleague in the next office to help me, but the words wouldn't come out properly. Eventually the ambulance came and I went to the hospital.

The doctor told me later that the stroke had damaged the blood supply to the right side of my brain, which controls the left side of my body. I had a CT scan, which showed that my stroke had been caused by a clot blocking one of the blood vessels in the brain and that, without a blood supply, the brain cells had died. Although all I felt like doing was lying in bed, the physical therapist explained that the quicker I got moving again, the greater the chance that the surviving nerve cells in my brain would remodel themselves to take over the actions of those that had died in the stroke.

TAY–SACHS DISEASE
An inherited condition that causes a child's brain to develop abnormally, and which is eventually fatal.

Children with Tay–Sachs disease lack a vital enzyme that is normally present in the brain. As a result, a harmful chemical that is normally broken down by this enzyme builds up in brain tissue and prevents some brain cells from developing normally. The disease becomes apparent at about five months old; until then an affected child appears to be developing normally. Parents may then notice that the child fails to develop any further skills and gradually loses head control and muscle tone. The diagnosis is confirmed by a blood test. There is no cure, and the disease is usually fatal by the age of five years. Tay–Sachs disease develops only if both parents carry a particular abnormal gene—even then, only one in four of their children is likely to be affected. The gene, and hence the condition, is most often found in Ashkenazi Jews and French Canadians. Screening for the abnormal gene is recommended for people in these high-risk groups who are planning a family.

TICS
Brief twitchy movements, most commonly occurring around the eyes, face, and neck.

Most mild tics start during childhood and disappear without treatment, often during adolescence. They usually involve a brief muscle spasm, which may be visible as twitching around the eyes or mouth or as a shoulder-shrugging motion.

Tics are also the main symptom of a distressing disorder known as Tourette's syndrome, which has a genetic component. The symptoms of this condition can be more disturbing and include muscular spasms and vocal outbursts that vary from simple grunts or throat clearing to words or sentences. Repeating what has just been said and the involuntary utterance of obscenities sometimes occur. The symptoms of Tourette's syndrome tend to wax and wane and are often at their worst during puberty. The spectrum of severity of the disease is very wide, ranging from almost unnoticeable to severely socially disabling. People with severe Tourette's syndrome usually need long-term drug therapy to suppress muscle spasms and often require specialist educational input.

TREMORS
A trembling or quivering movement of one or more parts of the body.

If we stretch our arms out, most of us will notice a slight tremor in our hands. This tremor often worsens with increasing age, at times of stress, or after too much caffeine or alcohol. Often, tremor is a symptom of an overactive thyroid gland, Parkinson's disease, or certain diseases of the cerebellum—the part of the brain that controls balance and movement. One fairly common condition, known as essential tremor, often runs in families. It can start at any age but usually becomes evident around 35 to 45 years of age. In this condition, the tremor affects both arms, although one is usually worse than the other. In a few people, essential tremor is so disabling that even basic activities such as writing, shaving, and holding a cup without spilling its contents become very difficult.

How is it diagnosed?
A doctor will try to establish the type of tremor and its specific cause by taking a medical history (p. 98) and performing a physical examination (p. 100).

What are the treatment options?
If the tremor is proved to be a symptom of another condition, then the doctor will give appropriate treatment. Mild essential tremor does not necessarily need treatment, especially if it is not causing disability or embarrassment. Severe, disabling symptoms can be reduced by drugs called beta-blockers or a particular anticonvulsant drug. In some people, the tremor responds to alcohol. Neurosurgery is a newer option, and even very severe tremor can be cured by procedures that disrupt a small part of the brain. Two methods are available: Either a small hole can be made in part of the brain, or an electrical stimulator wire can be left in the brain, and connected to a battery and control unit under the skin of the chest, much like a heart pacemaker.

TUMORS
Growths, either benign or malignant, that develop in the brain or spinal cord.

Although many brain tumors are not cancerous, they all need specialist attention, because they can press on brain tissue and increase the pressure inside the skull. Spinal tumors are very rare but they too can press on the spinal cord and lead to paralysis. The growths that originate in the brain or spinal tissue are known as primary tumors and those that have spread from other parts of the body, usually the lung, breast, ovary, or as a complication of some skin and blood cancers, are called secondary tumors. There are several types of primary tumor: Gliomas are the most common and develop from the nerves themselves; meningiomas are benign tumors composed of cells from the meninges, the protective membranes around the brain and spinal cord; neuromas are benign tumors of the spine.

What are the causes?
Experts do not fully understand under what conditions primary brain and spinal tumors develop. Secondary tumors spread via either the bloodstream or lymphatic system, or they infiltrate the brain directly from nearby areas such as the nose or face.

What are the symptoms?
Many of the symptoms of a tumor depend on the area of the brain or the level of the spine affected. For example, someone with a tumor in the part of the brain responsible for movement may experience weakness in the limbs. Other

symptoms, though, are caused by the increase of pressure within the skull. Generally the symptoms of a brain tumor include the following:

- Seizures
- Weakness in the limbs, loss of vision, or difficulty speaking
- Headaches, which may be worse in the morning and when stooping or coughing
- Nausea and vomiting
- Drowsiness
- Personality changes

If the tumor is in the spinal cord, a person may have back pain and a gradual weakness or loss of limb sensation.

How is it diagnosed?

If, from the medical history and physical examination (p. 98), a doctor suspects a tumor, computed tomography scanning (p. 106) or magnetic resonance imaging (p. 108) will probably be arranged to take a close look at the brain or spinal cord. It is important that the doctor establishes whether the tumor is a primary or secondary growth, especially as this decision will influence whether other parts of the body, such as the lungs, should be checked for cancer. Sometimes, a small piece of the tumor is removed during an operation called a craniotomy (p. 125) and examined under a microscope.

What are the treatment options?

Often the entire tumor, or certainly a large part of it, can be removed by surgery (p. 122). Meningiomas are easier than most to remove, but tumors that grow from the brain cells themselves are more difficult to remove completely. These tumors may be treated by a combination of laser surgery and radiotherapy. Secondary tumors are usually treated with a combination of drugs, chemotherapy, and radiotherapy.

VIRAL ENCEPHALITIS

This condition affects the brain tissue, which becomes inflamed as a result of a viral infection.

The viruses that can lead to encephalitis include those ones that cause mumps and measles (although these are rare since effective vaccination programs) and the herpes simplex virus, which causes cold sores. These viruses enter the body through the nose or mouth and then spread to the brain via the bloodstream or along the nerves.

What are the symptoms?

The symptoms vary widely and depend on which virus has caused the inflammation and the strength of the person's immune system. Usually, encephalitis develops as a complication of another viral illness, and the first symptoms are headache, fever, and drowsiness. The most severe type of encephalitis is generally caused by the herpes simplex virus, which induces the affected person to appear confused and behave in an unusual manner. Depending on the areas of the brain affected, limb weakness, speech difficulty, and seizures may develop.

How is it diagnosed?

Often the doctor will suspect that a person has encephalitis on the basis of a physical examination and a description of the symptoms. Brain imaging using computed tomography scanning (p. 106) or magnetic resonance imaging (p. 108) will usually reveal any swelling.

Different viruses affect different areas of the brain, so identifying the site of swelling is helpful. A sample of cerebrospinal fluid is usually removed during a spinal tap (p. 103), and sometimes the responsible virus shows up in the fluid—this generally takes one to two weeks. In some cases, an electroencephalogram (p. 111) is used to look at the electrical activity in the brain, and very occasionally a brain biopsy (p. 112) is necessary.

What are the treatment options?

Most cases of viral encephalitis are mild, and people recover spontaneously. Herpes simplex encephalitis, however, is more serious and needs treatment in a hospital with an intravenous drug called aciclovir for about ten days. Aciclovir stops the virus from replicating and causing further brain damage. If a person is having seizures, anticonvulsant drugs will be given to prevent them. Expert nursing care is required, and sometimes treatment in an intensive care unit may be necessary. Following recovery from severe encephalitis, a person may be left with some disability and will need rehabilitation, either at home or in a rehabilitation center.

What is the outlook?

Many people with mild encephalitis recover fully without needing treatment. Encephalitis caused by the herpes simplex virus can be very serious and is fatal in about one in five cases. Although the vast majority of people recover, they may not make a full recovery, and about one-third will have problems with memory, speech, or epileptic seizures.

Index

Acknowledgments

Carroll & Brown Limited would also like to thank:

Editorial assistant
Charlotte Beech

Picture researcher
Richard Soar

Production manager
Karol Davies

Production controller
Nigel Reed

Computer management
Elisa Merino, Paul Stradling

Indexer
Kathy Croom

3-D anatomy
Mirashade/Matt Gould

Illustrators
Andy Baker, Susan Doyle, Debbie Maizels, Gillian Martin, Mikki Rain

Photographers
Jules Selmes, David Murray

Photographic sources
6 (*left*) Quest/SPL
7 Cecil H. Fox/SPL
8 (*top*) CNRI/SPL
10 (*right*) S. Miller, Custom Medical Stock Photo/SPL
11 (*top*) GettyOne Stone
11 (*bottom*) Petit Format/ Nestlé/SPL
12 (*bottom*) Dr. Don Fawcett/SPL
13 (*top*) Mike Agltolo/SPL
14 (*right*) CNRI/SPL
15 Eye of Science/SPL
16 (*right*) Telegraph Colour Library
19 (*top*) Quest/SPL
19 (*bottom*) The Stock Market
20 GJLP-CNRI/SPL
21 Pictor
22 (*top*) Eye of Science/SPL
22/3 Quest/SPL

32 (*top*) GettyOne Stone
(*bottom*) Telegraph Colour Library
34 (*top*) Telegraph Colour Library
34 (*bottom*) Damasio H, Grabowski T, Frank R, Galaburda AM, Damasio AR: The Return of Phineas Gage: Clues about the brain from a famous patient. Science, 264:1102-1105, 1994. Department of Neurology and Image Analysis Facility, University of Iowa
34/5 GJLP-CNRI/SPL
36/7 The Stock Market
40 Dr. John Mazziotta et al/SPL
43 The Stock Market
47 www.floatworks.com
48 (*left*) GettyOne Stone
49 The Stock Market
50 (*centre*) Telegraph Colour Library
(*top right*) GettyOne Stone
(*bottom right*) The Stock Market
53 Telegraph Colour Library
56 (*top*) GettyOne Stone
60 GettyOne Stone
61 (*right, centre above*) Telegraph Colour Library
63 GettyOne Stone
65 (*top*) www.floatworks.com
66 (*bottom left*) Image Bank
(*bottom right*) Telegraph Colour Library
68 (*centre*) Telegraph Colour Library
(*top left, top right*) Image Bank
73 (*top*) Image Bank
73 (*bottom*) GettyOne Stone
77 (*bottom*) Sally Greenhill
80 (*left, centre bottom*) Image Bank
85 (*bottom*) Images Colour Library
86 GettyOne Stone
88 (*top left*) Gary R. Bonner
(*centre left*) Images Colour Library
(*centre right*) Image Bank
(*right*) Images Colour Library
91 (*centre left*) Images Colour Library
92 (*left*) Cecil H. Fox/SPL
(*centre*) Corbis

(*right*) Juergen Berger, Max-Planck Institute/SPL
93 Jerry Mason/SPL
96 Cecil H. Fox/SPL
97 Sean O'Brien/SPL
99 (*left*) Mehau Kulyk/SPL
(*centre*) BSIP Boucharlat/SPL
(*right*) Alfred Pasieka/SPL
101 Juergen Berger, Max-Planck Institute/SPL
102 (*top*) Simon Fraser/SPL
(*bottom*) Eye of Science/SPL
103 (*top*) CNRI/SPL
104 Department of Clinical Radiology, Salisbury District Hospital/SPL
105 (*left*) CNRI/SPL
(*top right*) CNRI/SPL
(*bottom right*) BSIP Dr. T. Pichard/SPL
106/7 Telegraph Colour Library
(*top left*) Alfred Pasieka/SPL
(*top right, bottom*) GCa/CNRI/ SPL
108 Image Bank
109 (*top*) Wellcome Trust Medical Photographic Library
(*bottom*) Alfred Pasieka/SPL
110 Geoff Tompkinson/SPL
111 (*left*) Jerry Mason/SPL
(*right*) BSIP VEM/SPL
112 Medipics
115 (*left*) Custom Medical Stock/SPL
117 Alfred Pasieka/SPL
118 BSIP Vem/SPL
121 Prof. P. Motta/G. Macchiarelli/ University 'La Sapienza' Rome/SPL
123 Pictor
124 (*top*) Kevin O'Neill
125 Kevin O'Neill
126 (*centre*) Simon Fraser/SPL
(*bottom*) Corbis
126/7 Corbis
127 (*top, centre left, bottom*) Corbis
(*centre right*) Kevin O'Neill
128 Kevin O'Neill
129 Images Colour Library

Back cover (*right*) Wellcome Trust Medical Photographic Library

160

619–001–2